DISCLAI

Cancer

The problem and the solution

Dr. Johanna Budwig

Translation:
Sprachendienste Holtz-Stosch GmbH
www.ho-st.de

ISBN 3-9810502-1-5

Original:
Krebs - das Problem und die Lösung
Sensei Verlag Kernen / Germany
www.sensei.de

Nexus GmbH Germany
Cannstatterstr. 13
71394 Kernen
www.nexus-book.com

JOHANNA BUDWIG, Dr. licenced pharmacist, qualified chemist, and with doctorates in chemistry and physics was senior expert for pharmaceuticals and fats in a high government function. She also studied medicine in order to implement the findings in the area of biochemistry of fats, in biophysical terms. The statements about "essential fats" or the "life threatening effects" of certain fats and their significance for the cancer problem lead to a collision with the prevailing opinion and to breaking off her medical studies. Convinced of her scientific findings on the natural science level, Dr. Budwig devoted her whole life for more than 50 years to the realization of the validity of her research results for sustaining human life in medicine, and in the process bring about a change in the direction of cancer research and therapy.

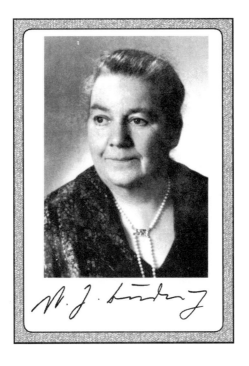

Contents:

Foreword to the 1st English edition

Dr. Johanna Budwig is rightly known far beyond the borders of Germany. Her ingenious, simple, and effective oil-protein diet has found adherents throughout the world and it has helped many people to particularly better deal with their cancer illness.

I had the great good fortune of spending many days in discussion with her over a period of several years, of being able to study her extensive case histories, of giving joint presentations with her, and of thus gaining an understanding of 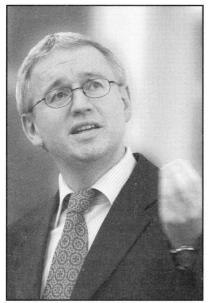 nutrition for myself that extended far beyond that which I was previously able to find in the usual literature. But what was most convincing to me in my activity on the executive board of *Cancer21* in Germany was the oil-protein diet. Hardly a day goes by when I do not talk with people on the phone who have changed their diet along the guidelines provided by Dr. Budwig. I am party first-hand to how successful this nutrition therapy is. I consciously use the term nutrition therapy and not cancer diet because I think it would be an injustice to Dr. Budwig to not to distinguish her scientifically grounded oil-protein therapy from all the diets that are offered around the world.

For me the oil-protein diet always serves as the basis of a cancer therapy and please understand that I am not just simply writing this, but that I have carefully chosen my words, as I have become familiar with more than 100 different alternative cancer therapies in recent years, and I have investigated many of them. When Dr. Johanna Budwig died the cancer scene lost one of the last great scientists of the last century, and it behooves each of us to carry her legacy to future generations, so that they as well can profit from the oil-protein diet.

Lothar Hirneise
www.hirneise.de

Introduction

The process of writing this book can truly be likened to a difficult birth. This delayed its publication date.

"Modern quantum physics - the rainbow over cancer research and cancer therapy", this is what this book is about. That was the content of my presentation in Freudenstadt, which was held in the Kurhaus on March 3rd 1999. Now it is not the quantum physics involved in successful cancer therapy and prevention that causes understanding difficulties. The citizen with average intelligence, yes I would say every reader can feel where truth prevails. This is also what Werner Heisenberg, quantum physicist noticed. The famous quantum physicist Max Planck emphasized: "When someone thinks he has discovered something new, but he cannot as a scientist so express it that everybody understands, then he hasn't discovered anything new at all."

I referred to this statement in my presentation in March 1999 in Freudenstadt. The reponse to my presentation in Freundenstadt confirmed this sentiment. This basis was undersood. I emphasized that I was not speaking about what caused the flood. I only speak about what the rainbow might be and what the dove with the olive leaf in its beak proclaims: There is land in sight. The activities of those, who in their supposed building declared themselves for solely authoritative, I did not mention.

Now very quickly as early as April 1999 activities were invoked by these representatives of chemotherapy and the champions of industrialy manufactured heated oils, which I reject. With "experts" and "authorities" the courts were brought in with "she said"!

It is my conviction that this dispute which these experts have invoked will contribute to the breakthrough of the better therapy for cancer patients and for better prevention.

This book, which also communicates the findings based on quantum physics, also contributes to mastery of the problems cited here. It is written in an understandable manner to serve an aid in understanding this problem.

The documentation will provide a good service in this regard.

The interview

Lothar Hirneise conducted this interview in 1998.

LH: What is the fundamental concept of your therapy?

JB: I was senior expert for pharmaceuticals and fats in the Federal Health Office; this was the highest authority in our country responsible for deciding on approvals for medication. At this time, 1951, many applications had been submitted to me for approval, or to be more precise, these were medications for cancer therapy with the sulfhydryl group (sulfur-containing protein compounds). Everywhere I saw that fats played a role, also in expert reports provided by well-known professors like Prof. Nonnenbruch.

Unfortunately, we could only detect fats in the late stage, and there were no chemical values to detect fats chemically at all. By this time, 1951, I had already developed the first chemical verifications for fat, jointly with Professor Kaufmann, the director of the German Federal Institute for Research on Grain, Potatoes and Fat, and my former doctoral advisor, who was also director of the Pharmaceutical Institute. This was published in 1950 in Neue Wege in der Fettforschung (New Directions in Fat Research).

Using the method of paper chromatography, which I had developed, I could analyze 0.1 mg of fat, and characterize it as highly unsaturated or unsaturated. We then published this extensively.

These were the first studies that made it even possible to detect linoleic acid or linolenic acid. Due to the importance of this work, 16 doctoral candidates were assigned to support my efforts. In this situation I noticed the sulfhydryl groups in my appraisal of the medications for cancer therapy. Through official channels I had the right to ask the companies questions relative to how they wanted to substantiate how this substance (sulfhydryl group) could help with cancer. The companies e.g. the company Knoll, which wanted to use these types of medications as cancer therapy were prepared to send all the copies of the created file, on my request.

Consequently, in early 1951, I got a very fast overview of where the problems were in this issue. That was the same year that B. Flaschenträger's manual appeared: Physiologische Chemie (Physiological Chemistry). The problem of automatic oxygen absorption for the living substrate is one of the most elementary questions in all of physiology, and it is one of the darkest. Everybody knows the sulfur-containing protein compound of the sulfhydryl group can be detected in all breathing tissues.

However another partner must be present in the interplay with this sulfhydryl group, because the self-active oxygen consumption in the living system is executed in a zig zag curve. Strictly speaking, it is manifest that oxygen consumption does not produce a reaction product; rather it occurs in an interplay between the positive electrically-charged sulphur compounds in the protein, and some kind of fatty substance that we cannot detect, because no verifications for it are available. This fatty substance however plays a major role in the Warburg's respiratory enzyme.

Warburg recognized that with the Warburg respiratory enzyme or the cytochrome oxydase, fats play a role in the lack of oxygen consumption and oxygen utilization (utilization in the living substrate). He wanted to overcome this

11

blockade in the experiment with butyric acid. This attempt was a failure.

LH: Does this mean that Warburg was the first who attempted to introduce more oxygen into the cell with butyric acid?

JB: No, von Helmholz, the man who discovered ozone, had attempted to get more oxygen into the cell. He showed that when we treat doves who have become asphyctic (i.e. doves that have been fed in such a manner that oxygen absorption is blocked), with increased ozone or oxygen, they then die more quickly – and this is still the case today. If the "oxygen bomb" is set up in the hospital for a person with oxygen deficiency, then the sick person dies more quickly.

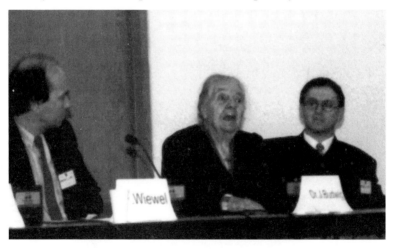

March 1999 / Freudenstadt-Germany
Frank Wiewel - People against Cancer USA
Dr. Johanna Budwig
Lothar Hirneise

If animals can be made asphyctic through a certain diet, e.g. bleached rice, then they suffocate and neither increased introduction of oxygen nor activation with any other possible substance will help. At this time we already knew vitamin A, B, C, D, and E, but this did not help. Prof. Linus Pauling for example had been involved with animal experiments and knew precisely that it had been published in 1951 that all vitamins had been investigated in searching for the respiratory activator for Warburg's respiratory enzyme, but this had produced absolutely nothing, not even vitamin C. By the way Professor Pauling, who had requested all my books from me personally, and who also received them from me, never referred to my work later.

And then the idea occurred to Warburg in 1926 that fats play a role. However he did not know which ones, and experimented with butyric acid. By the way, [Albert] Svent György also experimented with fats and wrote as early as 1952 that the substances are too easily oxidized and we cannot detect them. In this situation I then published my new ways of fat analysis, namely to introduce sensitive and specific verifications, nice stains. I was able to analyze fats precisely and break them down into the individual fatty acid components.

LH: What effects do these fatty acids have?

JB: They form the opposite electrical pole to the positively charged protein in the cell nucleus. They are located in the cell membrane and have been known for a long time as lipoids (fatty substances). In the case of tumor formation it was not known why cells in division are present in such great quantities. The wrong concept is still being pursued in medicine today; the tumor is associated with too much growth. This is incorrect. In 1956, I had published that with the tumor many cells in division are present, and amitosis has already started (see Fig.).

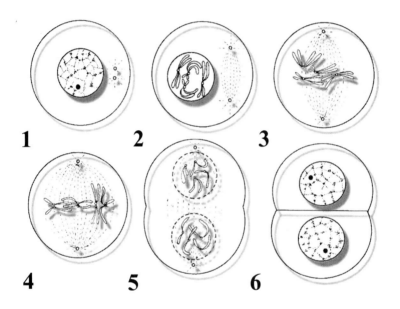

However in the case of tumor formation, cleavage of the daughter cell is lacking, which then results in rejection of the aging cells. When a leaf falls from a tree, a skin has formed over it and this vital function for normal the growth process is interrupted if the electrically charged fatty acids are lacking.

LH: How are fatty acids charged electronically?

JB: An important physicist, Kenneth Ford, said in 1966 that the elementary function of the electron exchange with the photons of solar energy is so intense, that one gets the impression the electrical energy stored in the electrons of seed oils, for example, still recognizes the relationship to its forbears in the photons of solar energy. Physically this has been strictly proven. And this absorption of solar energy in seeds is already adjusted in the green leaf to certain very specific wavelengths; science refers to this via the quantosomes. The quanta of physics, of the wave movement are adjusted to the photons of solar energy. This means that they do not even absorb other rays, and if other radiation such as with the transport of nuclear waster (1998) influences human functions, the elementary function between fats and proteins for oxygen absorption, then the radiation from the ashes of the atom bomb work so radically that this dipolarity which must remain in interplay in movement for the life process, is torn apart and the life function is destroyed. In physics these products in physical processes that disturb (i.e. pull apart) the dipolarity in the life process, which really should be banned, have been called radicals for a long time.

Now if you expose a normal life function, regardless of whether it is a seed or a person, to these rays, then intervention in the life function is so radical that in these experiments with quanta biology with the wrong rays even rats and mice jump around until they fall to the floor dead. The term radical comes from physics and was later used as camouflage for the highly heated oils, which we do not want to name by name, but that work exactly the same way. The base reaction of oxygen consumption and energy extraction from food is executed in the interplay of positive sulfur-containing protein, electronically highly charged with the photons that are suitable in terms of solar energy quanta, stored in seed oils of various quality. This dipolarity differs in quality and it is crucial for the function of the fatty acids that are recognized as vital. Other fatty acids that have a shorter fatty acid chain, e.g. 4, 6, or 8 links, are also utilized under other conditions in the life process.

Here however we are only referring to the fatty acids that are recognized as vital with 18 links in the hydrogen chains (chain with 18 links) and with high electronic enhancement. It is scientifically known that the electronic energy, e.g. in the linoleic fatty acids, is so high-grade that this energy lifts off of the heavy mass and moves as an electron cloud. You must start with the idea that heavy matter, charged positively, pulls down, the electrons pull upwards. In this dipolarity man can stand up, and in this dipolarity man has more capacity to store solar photons than does any other form of life, as demonstrated in the quantum biology of Professor Dessauer in 1954. It is particularly in the brain that these electrons are highly enhanced.

LH: What is an electron cloud?

JB: If the enhancement of electronic energy is always higher through absorption of photons in the electron compounds of the fats, then the power of the electrons is so high in the dipolarity in between gravity and electrons, that they move from the fatty acid, (which also contains hydrogen compounds, and which is heavy matter), over the chain with electrons.

LH: What is the significance of the cloud?

JB: No life form has as much energy to store the electrons and photons in depots as does man. This electronic energy, stored in the electronic substrate of the human being, stored particularly in the vital, highly unsaturated fatty acids, is such a strong life element for man, that it was correctly said previously that these are certain fatty acids that have been recognized as vital foodstuffs. Man cannot live without them.

For instance, chemists measure the iodine value of fats and say that if oils have a certain iodine value, then these oils are unsaturated. If oils, regardless of whether sunflower oil or flax oil, are treated with overheated steam then these oils can indeed give a positive iodine value, but they are not the vital fats with 18 links, but rather they form cross-links between the fatty acids like a large net, and are highly detrimental to metabolism of the fats, and with protein they act like radicals.

I repeat because it is so important: I have detected particles in oils treated with steam, which indeed have a positive iodine value, but which are highly toxic for man.

LH: And you attempt to avoid this toxin when treating people who are sick?

In my nutrition therapy I expressly switch off these fats. By the way the discovery of switching-off these toxic oils, has been recognized as nationally worthwhile since 1971. In the oil and fat industry production has not been changed to this day, because they say these products are billion-dollar items, and nobody will give the industry money to establish something new. That is understandable. The representatives of chemotherapy pose another problem. Our chemotherapy is aimed at destruction of the tumor, and it is recognized that chemotherapies destroy many living cells, and the entire person. Anything that disturbs growth is fatal because growth, as elementary life function, is part of the life process of man. We cannot achieve something good with bad tools.

LH: Can you tell us something more about the unsaturated fatty acids and their net-like connections?

JB: For a moment try to forget everything that you have read previously. In butter the fatty acids consist of 4 carbon compounds, in coconut fat, goat fat, and sheep fat the fatty acids consist of 6, 8, 10, or 12 carbon compounds respectively. The unsaturated vital fatty acids really start in the chain with 18 carbon compounds. For example, in olive oil there is only one unsaturated bond in the fatty acid. A person who has a deficiency of vital fats does not absorb it. Thus today's publicity concerning olive oil does not help at all. The fatty acid chains are primarly saturated in the lower area of the carbon chain links, butyric acid, coconut fat, and palm fat, primarily saturated, however they are more easily co-combustible for people if the essential fatty acids are present. The fatty acids with 18 links are the most important essential fatty acids. There are also fatty acids with up to 30 links.

Fatty acids with 18 links, like in sunflower oil or in flax oil with the higher level of unsaturation, are more important for people, particularly for the brain functions of man.

The carbon compounds are heavy matter, even in the fatty acid. If two people reach out to each other with two arms, then they are more strongly bound to each than if they only extend one arm. It is precisely the same for carbon. The fatty acid in olive oil is not considered to be a vital fatty acid; it can only be co-combusted in the organism if essential fatty acids are also present. Linoleic acid rich in electrons is considered vital. There is a particularly high amount of energy in this double double bond of the linoleic acid. This energy wanders and is not fixed in place as it is with a chemical compound, such as with table salt.

This energy, wandering between electrons and the positively charged protein with sulfhydryl groups is an alternating association process in the electromagnetic field. This is very important. Perhaps you are familiar with the painting of Michelangelo, where God creates Adam (two fingers pointing to each other, however they do not touch). This is quantum physics, the fingers do not touch. The physicists who I know, Max Planck, or Albert Einstein, or Professor Dessauer all represent the view that man is created by God in His image. You see in being together as human beings there is certainly also a connection without directly touching the other person. People who maintain that they only believe what they can touch are wrong.

The dipolarity with a simple double bond in olive oil is weaker than it is in sunflower seed oil, which is bonded twice. This double double bond is considered to be vital for man. However if the same chain length of 18 carbons has three unsaturated fatty acid compounds, then the electrical energy is as strong as a magnet, depending on the position of the double bond. If double combinations are now closer together, then the energy is greater. All electrical energy that is in movement produces a current that flows and spreads a magnetic field. These electrons also have a magnetic field. You can see this on the window when it rains, for instance. When one drop comes down, it attracts another drop and becomes a larger drop. Precisely the same principle applies with electrons.

This electronic energy is negatively charged. The positively charged sulfhydryl groups of the protein adhere in the unsaturated bonds where the electrons are and that is where they insert their sulphur-containing compounds.

This produces the lipoproteins. The life process is sustained in the interplay between the positively-charged particles and negatively-charged particles. In this process there is no connection, and this is our life element. If a radical break occurs at this point through fatty acids that no longer give off electronic energy, but rather are cross-linked like a net, then the dipolarity can no longer work actively in this net. This is the deadly effect of radicals, because instead of the chains with the electron clouds they interlace a net without electron clouds, indeed with unsaturated bonds, but without dipolarity. I quickly knew that the triple unsaturated fatty acids, which were called linolenic acid, and which no one had isolated before me, had 18 links and that they did not always carry their double bonds at the same point.

They have such a strong electronic energy compared to the heavier matter in the 18-link fatty acid chains, that biologically this energy is far greater than it is with the next arachidon acid with 20 links. The highest electron collection is with the combination of linoleic-linolenic fatty acids in flax oil. The linolenic acid as conjugated (interaction of neighboring double bonds in the molecule that are separated by a single bond) fatty acid is even more effective and is even more strongly effective in interplay with linoleic acid as it is present in the flax oil chain as essential fatty acids for oxygen absorption. This was relatively easy for me to verify in my experiments. I would like to emphasize this. The combination of double unsaturated linoleic acid with triple unsaturated linolenic acid is particularly well-combined in flaxseed. Naturally the quality of flaxseed differs greatly. Naturally red flowering flaxseed and blue flowering flaxseed are naturally different; there is also a difference depending on whether flaxseed is harvested in the cold like in Siberia, or in Africa.

LH: Is it this energy that heals cancer?

JB: Yes, this energy is now movable and it is easily released. It is precisely this energy that heals cancer, or does not even allow it to occur. If this vital element is present then no tumor can occur. This vital element is a deciding factor in the immune system. There is a lot of talk these days about immune defense. There is no effective factor in the immune system other than the essential fatty acids. Let's take for example a patient with a breast tumor. I do not radiate the woman directly on the tumor with my laser, rather I soak the surrounding tissue with fat and protein through the diet, use my oils, e.g. ELDI oils for external application, and radiate the healthy tissue.

Another case. For example I had a child here with a sarcoma in the bone. The child repeatedly claimed that somebody pushed him in kindergarten and he fell on a sharp rock. Since then I have had this. The doctors say, that's nonsense, falling on a sharp rock does not cause a sarcoma. But I say, if the child's immune system is weak, and the child is injured, then this can be a trigger.

LH: But shouldn't all those people who eat these heated oils get cancer?

JB: It is very important to view the person as a unit consisting of body, soul, and psyche. However, the factor that is primarily effective at the moment can be quite different. I am still convinced today that if a woman has a very poor marriage, and has to deal with suppression and taunts from her husband day in and day out, then I cannot help her with quark-flax oil. All three factors belong together in a human person. Here is another example. It is very cold here in November. Let's assume that several people must spend the night outdoors. One takes a hot bath and everything is fine. Another gets lymphogranulomatosis, and another gets pneumonia. They do not all get sick in the same way. The life function of the person always plays a very significant role.

Or let's look at another case. I have a patient with lung metastases. Her doctor from Ulm came along as well. I counseled her first to change the diet, and then use the oil pack with ELDI oils, to more quickly dissolve the metastasis. The patient was rubbed with oils over the entire body, but naturally in determining the diet and the environment, the whole person must be taken into consideration. This patient knew that she had been given up on. I set up the diet in different steps. Now the patient lives in Ulm and against my advice, she is involved with yoga.

In this case I counseled against yoga, and recommended autogenic training, so that her body is pacified and her body is balanced and calm. Often yoga or sport is very important, but sometimes the patient should not do this. Guiding the sick person is very important. There is no one treatment that applies for everyone. The patient must also feel for himself what is good for him. Yoga alone cannot replace the healthy basis of nutrition.

LH: Does this mean that generally you do not recommend physical training?

JB: Correct, it must always be viewed individually. I would never allow a cancer patient with metastases to jog, ride a bicycle, or to practice yoga. His body must relax. I am more an adherent of Zen philosophy in this area. It is based very much on the factor: Let it come. Do not be inactive, rather be very active. I activate in my consulting, the patient should not stay in bed, stretch out and let others act. That is incorrect. The patient must work as well. On the other hand, unfortunately I have often experienced what it means when family members do not participate, for example if food is prepared without love, and if the family member basically rejects the treatment. The whole subject of sport must be treated on a very individual basis.

LH: Do you think that a large tumor must be operated on.

JB: I can't make a general statement here. I totally reject radiation and chemo; I also reject hormonal treatment for abdominal cancer. However, operations must be considered very individually. This also applies for tumors in the intestine. I am not a proponent of quickly creating an artificial anus. The ubiquitous technocracy no longer does justice to people.

LH: How did you get your homeopathic license?

JB: I acquired my insights in the area of natural science as a well trained expert for fats and pharmaceuticals in a responsible position. Then I tried to make my findings regarding the significance of the highly unsaturated fats and the damage caused by denatured fats known. Naturally this is not necessarily connected with the practice of homeopathy.

However as the number of sick people who sought and received help from me increased, the number of attacks from the medical fraternity who viewed my nutritional advice as an encroachment in their area also increased. Up to 1968, these attacks from doctors were unsuccessful. In 1968, I realized that the use of laser radiation is only possible if the resonance capability is provided in the biological area based on my quantum biological findings. In the USA it was published at that time that the absorption capacity in the living substrate must still be verified.

In this regard, I created the so-called ELDI oils (Electron Differentiation oils) through exact spectroscopic measurements via the absorption of light in different oils. This enabled me to immediately switch the metabolism to positive using the ruby laser that I had chosen. The success was surprising, even to me. These ELDI oils, which are used externally, have a very favorable retuning effect on the metabolism for people who are ill. With my knowledge of the borderline situation concerning the practice of alternative medicine, I said to myself, if I now treat with laser beams, then that constitutes treatment of sick people. Consequently, I obtained the additional permission to practice as a non-medical practitioner.

LH: But then you also studied medicine.

JB: That's right, in 1955 and in the following years, I also studied medicine, totally real with anatomy and everything that goes along with it. Through the illness of Ms. Martius (wife of the well-known Professor Martius in Göttingen, I am not revealing any unauthorized secret, because this was carried in all the press releases), where I was called on for advice, I was able to use my therapy in various clinics in Göttingen. This was very successful, as is documented in my book Der Tod des Tumors Bd. II (The Death of the Tumor Vol. II). Then, however, I reached a limit as industrial groups and also professors became involved.

Since the people who were opposed to what I was doing always said that I had not studied medicine, I took the time in Göttingen to study medicine. I still remember the time I was working late one night in Göttingen, a woman came to me, with her small child whose arm was supposed to be amputated due to a tumor (sarcoma). I told her what she should do and soon thereafter the subject of amputation was dismissed and the child quickly did very well.

Because I was still a medical student at this time, I was summoned to appear before the Municipal Court due to a petition that I should be prohibited from studying medicine. I was accused of walking through surgery clinics, looking for patients and pulling them out of the clinic. Then I said: "I have never been in the surgery clinic, I do not even know where it is," I explained that the mother sought me out; I did not seek her out.

I then asked what I should do. Shouldn't I help the child? Because I demonstrably helped a patient successfully (documented in the book Der Tod des Tumors Bd. II (The Death of the Tumor Vol. II), there was a petition to bar me from studying medicine. But the director of the court and counsel for the university, Dr. Henze, rejected this and said: "You have nothing to fear. In my area of jurisdiction nothing will happen to you. If it does there will be a scandal in the scientific community."

Nevertheless, I concluded that I could better deal with the opponents to my direction as a university graduate and no longer as student. And I still believe today that this decision was right.

LH: Where have you had the opportunity of presenting your position at congresses and presentations?

JB: A very important presentation was held in 1964 in the Hilton Hotel in Chicago, at the invitation of the American Oil Chemists Society. Before Professor Kaufmann and I published the validity of my finding concerning the significance of the highly unsaturated fats for the vital function of the human being, Dr. Kaufmann wanted to be sure, and he ordered cytochrome dyed yellow-green in vials from the company Mack in Illertissen. This is considered to be the preliminary stage for hemoglobin, the blood pigment that cancer patients do not produce adequately.

He gave me the yellow-green cytochrome on paper and said: "Touch this and see if it turns red." I touched it and it turned red, then Prof Kaufmann asked; "Do you have red paint on your finger?" I laughed and said, "No Professor, you can do the same thing as well. Touch it with your fingers." It turned red, and I said: "I know that you have now started eating flax oil, too." Then the audience stood up and applauded me. This presentation is in my book Kosmische Kräfte gegen

Krebs (Cosmic Powers Against Cancer). Another important presentation was given in Tokyo, where I was the first woman allowed to speak at a congress. At night in my hotel then several women requested that I should give a presentation on the role of women in the world because the newspapers were devoting a lot of attention to the fact that I was the first woman who had been allowed to speak at a conference.

That's why I was no longer impressed that German doctors who knew too little of real science criticized my work as all philosophy and not science, which is still going on to this day. However I have the impression that the public trend, recognizing the importance of the natural basis for the vital function of the human being, has also become so strong, even in Germany, that pure medical doctrine must join it. The German physician Dr. Roehm who immigrated to the USA published an article in the USA in favor of my work: Who are we, we doctors? In this article he takes the position that it is beneath the dignity of physicians to exclude the natural basis of the life function, as is still attempted in Germany to a great extent. By the way, on the advice of friends in Innsbruck I have put all my scientific work together in a well organized manner (see Presentations at congresses, see Appendix….).

LH: Does a cell become malignant if it does not get enough oxygen?

JB: There is an error in your question, because your question reduces the human being to a cell that is not possible. In humans the lymph system plays a very significant role in the metabolism of fats. When discussing this holistic medical issue you should not localize on the cell, but to return to my previous example – when this child falls on a sharp stone in kindergarten then the important thing is which immune forces are active in the body and which are not.

You see, a doctor comes to me with his 12-year-old child. As I said previously, I always let the sick person speak for himself, this applies to children as well. The boy was happy that he was now allowed speak and said: "OK, now I am going to tell you something. The man who is sitting over there is my father. But the woman sitting next to him is not my mother, that is his secretary, and my mother does not live with us. When my mother lives with us then the muesli tastes good. And when this woman makes the muesli, it doesn't taste good at all."

The father turned very red indeed. You see, these things are very important. You cannot reduce the illness to the cells. When people learn that they have been given up on by allopathy then I ask whether the patient is Catholic or Lutheran. And often the patients proceed to tell me for instance how much they are troubled by the fact that they have not been to confession for some time.

Then I tell the patients that before they return in 4 weeks, they should go to confession, and speak openly with their priest. I am Lutheran myself. I always take the whole person very seriously.

LH: What do you recommend when people do not want to eat quark for ideological reasons or because it does not agree with them?

JB: A well-known professor from Sweden who is director of a sanatorium for biological therapies, and who knows my treatment very well, called me because he had been called into treat President Bill Clinton and, according to his information, unfortunately President Clinton cannot eat quark. I did not give him any advice. But I can tell you the following. I have never had a patient who was not able to eat quark in combination with my oil-protein diet.

LH: What do you recommend to people as a preventative measure so that they don't get cancer at all?

JB: Only flax oil as oil. I reject all meat that is in the stores. Fresh meat is OK. Nothing from the frozen food section. You should bake your bread yourself. Oleolux, for example, is something that lasts longer than flaxseed that you can spread on bread or add to vegetables (see the instructions on the next page). You should also prepare your fruit juices yourself. Potatoes are OK, so is cheese.

Also the electromagnetic environment in which we live is very important. Also the textiles that we wear are not insignificant. I reject synthetic materials because they consume too many forces.

I dislike modern foam mattresses because they rob too much energy from you when you sleep. A lot of wood is important in home construction. Carpets are also important so that radiation remains as biological as possible. Gemstones and semi-gem stones are also important because they have good biological radiation and thereby they influence the environment. Books could be written about the favorable effects of gem stones. The environment and living conditions must be as biologic as possible. The lifestyle, e.g. regular sleep is very important. Many cancer patients stay up too late at night and sleep too long in the morning. There is often incorrect or misleading advertising on the labels of our grocery products.

There are hundreds of such aspects that must be taken into consideration. I would never maintain that I heal patients with tumors with the oil-protein diet, on the other hand I get a steady stream of confirmations of my work from recognized experts, that in the surgery clinic in Helsinki they have experienced a success rate of 90% and more, when using the findings of Dr. Budwig, and this success was achieved in cases where allopathy failed. This was submitted by Professor Halme.

LH: How do you work with patients?

JB: When patients come, I generally schedule two hours for the initial discussion; this is usually between 3:00 and 5:00 in the afternoon. Usually I let the patient report first – about his difficulties, treatments, diagnoses that he is aware of, the medical history, which therapeutic measures have been already employed, etc. In this report, I also learn about the patient's environment, the workplace, what kind of work the patient has done, and I also learn about the living conditions, e.g. condition of the marriage, and the diet.

After the first half hour, I then explain my position relative to the social/political situation. I explain that the trend in the German Medical Association of playing up the image of the physician is associated with a certain coercion that the physician may not use natural healing methods. For many years, Dr. Loeckle has resisted this coercion and the public discussion in this regard has been going on in the New Juristische Wochenscrift (official legal journal) since 1962 and has stayed there for many years, all under the heading, cancer therapy as a legal issue. After I briefly cite how I would go about my treatment in the specific case, then about

4:00 pm I give the patient and his family time to decide whether they want to follow the path I have outlined; indeed either whole-heartedly or not at all.

Partial treatment, in combination with my direction, by doctors who have too strict conditions against the use of natural healing is not possible. Until 1997 this was prohibited by the medical association, and consequently neither was this possible from my side. It was only in 1997 that the German Medical Association changed the Federal Medical Practitioners Act so that doctors could also use natural healing methods. If the patient then decides to use my advice, I become active step-by-step. I respond to the nutrition issues and my applications are documented in writing.

Since 1968 I have been using the ELDI oils extensively for external application for rubbing on the entire body, and for focused application of the oil pack or oil wraps. Where required I also use these ELDI oils rectally. What I prohibit is just as important as what I prescribe in my consultation. The products I mention have been produced in accordance with my discoveries and my activity as an inventor, to ensure the shelf life in these natural products, without the use of antioxidants and preservatives. This inventive activity also includes legally what is excluded from my side because, according to my findings, a more extensive complex of industrial processed fats is highly damaging to the vital function, and I consistently exclude this group of foodstuffs. Naturally, in this respect, the economic strategy but also the education of doctors are impacted by my advice and they are not always in agreement with that which I offer patients as assistance. Patients who come to me usually must return at 3 or 4-week intervals. They pay DM 1,000.00 for the 1st visit; likewise they pay DM 1,000.00 for the second and for the third visit. After that they don't pay anything, although sometimes they come regularly for more than 10 years. They can also call me daily between 6:00 and 8:00 pm, or they can get information per fax.

LH: Are there also patients who never return?

JB: Recently I have experienced an increased number of patients who want my advice and so-called preliminary information, and do not clearly state this. They want to learn as much as possible and then continue to be treated by their professor. Under this prerequisite, it is clear it is not particularly the poorest patients who come to me. For two years I advised old people and poor people at no charge, but this did not produce much because the social conditions in Germany are very complicated. If patients come to me who emphasize that they are thankful that they are financially and intellectually independent, then I also demand this engagement in the realization of my practice.

When people come who are seriously ill with cancer--for instance, members of parliament or other politicians from Bonn--who are confronted with the question of whether they should undergo chemotherapy, but want to continue being treated by their professor, because he says he wants to integrate my findings, this usually results in complications because in training and ability to reason this doctor is not capable of correctly evaluating the holistic behavior of my therapy.

A patient from Canada with a tumor on the pituitary gland was supposed to be treated with chemotherapy. With my therapy, I quickly had good success. When more pressure was exerted by the clinic to take the usual chemicals and medications that the clinic prescribed, he responded: "Dr. Budwig has a different philosophy. I will stay on this path." It depends on his capacity to decide and his independence from professors. Often the professors insist on their superior knowledge to the disadvantage of the patients.

LH: There are many questions about cardinal trace elements, acid base balance, free radicals, and vitamins being discussed today. What is your view of this discussion?

JB: In this regard, I emphasize that vitamins have been known for decades and are significant, likewise the acid-base balance and trace elements like selenium, germanium, and all the others. In 1951, in the search for a factor which was capable of re-stimulating the reduced oxygen balance in the biological milieu, the attempt was made to use the products just mentioned. This was not possible over the whole line. Neither trace elements nor vitamins were capable of regulating the function of the respiratory enzymes again.

There is another factor that I would particularly like to discuss. In 1952, after my scientific work was published, one scientist recognized the significance of the highly unsaturated fats very precisely. He came to Germany from the USA and returned to the USA. To protect the large companies, he simply named these substances radicals, which radically intervene in the intact function of the respiratory enzymes, without the doctors or the public understanding this.

This so-called "scientist" was to a large degree responsible for the erroneous trend, so then hundreds of other scientists attacked my quantum biological findings with everything in their vocabulary, but the one point which must be switched off, kept in darkness, namely the pseudo fats, fats that are not fats. One scientist in the USA, a professor of natural science published: "Our society is sacrificing itself on the altar of pseudo-science if it does not want to ultimately acknowledge what is being offered to people as edible fat. We cannot avoid this issue."

Fats are the substances that govern all life phenomena, which responsibly participate for orderly vital function, growth and absorption of the sun. Vitamins, trace elements etc. offer no aid to a person if he has been harmed by consuming the wrong fats. We must recognize the reason for the damage if we want to help this person. Many physicians have asked me after my presentations; "What about everything that we have learned. Is all that useless now?" I answered: "Everyone should do what he can."

Whether he cures with cold water, or with overheating baths, with psychology or via the psychiatrist, he can use everything. But it will all be of no avail to the person who has been affected in the foundation of his vital function, namely impairment of the consumption of oxygen and solar energy. This impairment of the basis of the vital function must be resolved. The dependence on the acid-base balance discussed so often today, this balance will only be restored if highly unsaturated fats are restored as the natural basis in the vital function in the blood and in the lymph of the person, through a natural supply of natural seed oils with the highly unsaturated fats. All other functions are important and remain important, but the base disturbance must be resolved.

LH: Which patients do you accept, or which ones would you not accept?

JB: I make a very clear distinction as to which patients I will still take and which patients I categorically will not accept. If cancer patients are full of metastases, the liver is involved, and the total condition is described as moribund (incurable) by the treating doctor, this does not bother me, I still accept these patients for treatment. I only take these patients if I am convinced, on the basis of the information available to me, that a good chance of healing through my treatment is present. I view the limit of my consulting for example in a patient for whom an artificial anus has been created, although I have had such a patient for more than 10 years.

I have been able to observe how often the stool excretions also go into the stomach area and we have had many operations performed. I cannot agree with this and be responsible for this with every patient. Thus I categorically do not accept patients for whom an artificial anus has been created. I also reject patients with breast cancer whose arm is already very swollen through water retention. The pain is too great because tumor masses have also collected behind the shoulder blade.

In this case, I do not accept the patient. I check the threshold very carefully. For example I have been able to achieve good success with brain tumors. I emphasize that of the patients who come to me, more than half of them are doctors and many are family members of doctors. My scientific successes, also due to the translation of my books, are known on all continents and consequently patients come from around the world. Currently (1998) I am treating patients from Hawaii, the USA, Africa, New Zealand, the Philippines,

Hong Kong, Canada, and from other countries. The efforts of good doctors to help my cause to breakthrough are underway throughout the world, particularly among Germans who have emigrated. I observe with the many physicians who have emigrated to the USA that they understand the suppression that I am subjected to here. I get a lot of affirmation from these doctors. For example, an oncologist in the USA who publicly did a lot to establish my cause was Dr. Roehm in Florida.

LH: How do sick people get off the track?

JB: For the most part, this has been explained in the previous responses. In their training doctors have only a very narrow education, not grounded in real science, and in this regard capital is highly effective. The preliminary mention of trace elements and vitamins etc. that are also important irritates patients unnecessarily. Patients come to me with handfuls of vitamins that do not help them, and which have only been prescribed through misleading advertising. Usually cancer patients are not helped in this manner.

LH: Where do you see the difficulty in getting physicians to think differently?

JB: Here the behavior of health insurance companies plays a major role, but I would say that the behavior of those doctors, not all doctors, who want get their money comfortably in accordance with the ritual prescribed by the guidelines of the insurance companies are not ready to relearn. But this has been the case in all ages, there have been good and bad representatives in all professions. Let's hope that the number of those who use your [my] knowledge with great responsibility will increase.

In this regard I consider a new direction in the USA to be very significant. It is called the Third Wave. This Third Wave which calls on the new elite is very well represented here in Germany as well. I learned about it from my patients and from teachers. In the Third Wave the opinion is that the elected representatives, particularly in the German parliament, no longer have the inclination, the time, nor the possibility to keep track of the flood of information that is coming forward from specialized areas, from the Internet for example. Now the politicians are called on, not only to listen to elected representatives or their experts for information, but also to add the genuine elite with knowledge and responsibility. I know for example that Mrs. Clinton in the USA also represents this cause. For example she helped get a few patients who I had treated get appointed to the health ministry. I am convinced that the new elite, with real knowledge and with real responsibility, is called on to stand up for true progress in medicine on all continents on the broadest basis possible. This primarily includes prevention. I agree with what Prof Jutta Limbach, president of the Federal Constitutional Court, published: "We can no longer remain a pure repair shop for bad policy. Politicians have their responsibility here to protect science and to support those who represent real progress, also against the power of large corporations."

LH: What would you say to politicians?

JB: If I were speaking to a politician who was honestly prepared to correct the large misappropriation of donations to politicians, then I would tell him that political influence through campaign funding donated by the major corporations must be terminated. Just think of the contributions involved in the political change of 1983. The issue in health administration, which is now highly current in 1998, must be approached differently. In other countries the natural direction is better supported by the government. One example of this is the University of Melbourne in Australia. The university has established the following new principles: All medical students must take classes in the colleges of chemistry and biochemistry each semester, and their professors must participate in the discussions in the colleges.

Cancer patients should be able to freely select the therapies they want. Patients must also be given the opportunity that the health insurance companies honor their obligation and finance the application of a natural therapy in the interest of patients.

LH: How come there are not enough natural scientists that support you?

JB: It is same with scientists as with most people, the Bible even says that everyone sought his own way. And there are very few people who are still willing to give all for their scientific findings. If they notice that the trend now is heading in this direction, then they want to be part of it. This is evidenced today by the publications on highly unsaturated fatty acids and their significance. The paper flood on highly unsaturated fatty acids or good plant oils and their significance for vital function is increasing.

However there is no concurrent mention as to what prevents this natural prerequisite. Dr. Williams, a physician from the Philippines who has very significantly published support of my cause, writes for instance in the Internet that with my publications unfortunately I have made myself an opponent of Unilever [major producer of fats]. He writes that these false fats are now contained in our daily products such as cakes, ready-to-eat food etc. There are even clinics that give out our flax oil in capsules. The directors of these clinics are even Noble Prize winners. While they indeed recognize how important flax oil is in the diet, they allow the other fats that we consume to go unnoticed.

Presentation in Frankfurt

Assigned discussion contribution 23.09.1998

Distinguished participants, I thank you for coming. The director of People Against Cancer, Mr. Frank Wiewel has just announced the program for this evening. You will hear something of the truth about cancer. I obligate myself to stick to this program. The well-known physicist, the quantum physicist, Max Planck, he is considered to be a theoretician among physicists, formulated the sentence: "When someone thinks he has discovered something new, but he cannot as a scientist so express it that everybody understands, then he hasn't discovered anything new at all." I maintain that I have discovered something new in the field of cancer therapy, which is of great consequence. The quantum physics, electrons interacting with solar energy in natural events is the crucial in this regard. I want to make things so clear to you that everyone here in this room who wants to listen for a half hour will also understand these things and after a half hour will no longer say, they are not believable.

A physician told me, "I understand only one thing about rainbows, they always dissappear when I want to touch them. This is correct. But there is an incorrect concept here. Even the physician can't get a hold of the rainbow and nature. Everybody, the doctor, the sick person who wants to be healthy, we are all part of nature. We must respect this fact. And it is the greatest physicists and quatum biologists who have reached the conclusion that we are created by God in his image, as Michelangelo so beutifully depicted in the creation of Adam.

Naturally there is no a miracle cure for cancer, however we will all recognize that people are involved. As long as a person lives, he must breathe, this you will agree with. And at this point the great scientist, Otto Warburg, in thorough work, determined that all tissue in the living organism, wherever a tumor can be formed, is characterized by the fact that it can no longer absorb oxygen. And at this point I had the good fortune, the blessing of working at the Federal Health Office responsible for the approval of medications, 1950 / 1951, to come to the awareness that the photo elements of life, the photons of the sun interacting with the electrons built up in the essential vital seed oils, are necessary for the absorption of oxygen. This is irrefutable.

The scientists who in 1951 sought for the deciding factor, the factor that would be capable of making the respiratory enzymes capable of functioning again, all knew that there was a substance, yellow-green and it is called cytochrome. This substance, which dominates in the blood of cancer patients, must be returned to the red blood red blood pigment.

Doctors say today that the blood forming pigments do not function correctly in patients with tumors who also have leukemia. This is correct. In this regard I would like to cite an experiment of decisive significance. Professor Kaufmann in Münster, director of the Pharmaceutical Institute, the Federal Institute for Fat Research and at the State Chemical Investigation Office where I worked, before we published the work, Untersuchung der Blutlipoide: Geschwulstproblem und Fettforschung (Investigation of Blood Lipoids: the tumor problem and fat research) organized an experiment. He ordered cytochrome, poured it on paper and said to me now show that it becomes red. I touched it and – it turned red. He looked at my hand: "Do you have red paint on your hands?" I said: "No professor you can do the same thing with your hands as well." He touched the paper and it turned red. Then I said: "I know that you have also started pouring flax oil in your yoghurt". This was the proof of the validity of my work: Ulcer problem and fat research. The lack of oxygen in tumor-bearing tissue was resolved.

The well-known physicist Professor Werner Heisenberg, described in his book how particularly in Germany, the ossified rigid thought processes of the adherents of the old school are always refuse to fully embrace new things. They always want to force the new into their old thought processes. That does not work! I still experience this today after 40 years. And Professor Heisenberg writes: "Even the suppression of new knowledge cannot prevent the breakthrough, because the people, the public, even if they are not experts in quantum physics or medicine, they have a feel for where truth rules.

I am convinced that most listeners will comprehend, in all the diversity which must still be taken into consideration, that there is an elementary factor for the recovery of people who are ill. The sick person must be able to absorb oxygen again. He must be able to breathe again. Naturally many factors are important here. However if we take a good look, then the protein in the cell nucleas is positively charged. The electrons in the peripheral of the cell – they oscillate in a cloud of electrons – represent the negative charge.

And in the middle energy oscillates uninterrupted in the electromagnetic field, which the electrons store from the photons of the sun in constant renewal, and always introduce anew into the life process. Now at the age of 90, I have the impression, that direction is establishing itself, very slowly but with great certainty. The growth promotion provided by electrons built up by the sun and stored in seed oils is important in overcoming the blockages in the tumor, which the obsolete scientists incorrectly fight with growth-inhibiting medications. The growth-inhibiting medications we currently use as chemotherapies are wrong. The energy produced by X-ray devices is also wrong, because it has a growth-inhibiting effect. Thus, if we want to use this elementary knowledge, we must take other factors into consideration, factors concerning proper respiration and restoration of the electromagnetic field in the metabolism of human beings, factors such as what the environment is like, what the opportunity for sleep is like, the issue of whether with plastics much too much vital energy is being withdrawn.

This is self-evident. Good juice, good food. However everything that starts with "anti-biological" is very suspicious. I read in the newspaper today that now there is to be a sudden entry in the area of nutrition for functional diet. I am convinced that the industry certainly knows, that it has been proven for a long time that the highly unsaturated vital fats in seed oils cannot be synthetically manufactured, nor can vitamin C, that is supposed to be function, be synthetically manufactured, nor can vitamin E that is supposed to be functional be synthetically manufactured. This is why rethinking on the part of the large corporations is required, and they have been aware of this for a long time.

In 1968 when information was published in America indicating that you cannot treat cancer patients with lasers because the burn damage is too great, that patients die within a few days, I thought about this statement and recalled that we certainly have absorbtion measurements in oils as an analysis method in the Federal Institute for Fat Research. I put oils together according to mathematic calculations of wave lengths and was given a laser device by Mr. von Siemens, a ruby laser. And Mr. Peter Siemens said to me: "How did you come to use this laser? This is the only one that reflects the light of the moon." I used this laser device in conjunction with the oils, for which I had calculated the absorbtion bands in the same wave range. And these oils have very successful for many many cancer patients since 1968. We also have a person in this room who used my therapy for his wife. I will not mention names but he lives here in Frankfurt. His wife was deathly ill and had even recieved an artificial vertrbrae; the wound did not heal so well, and now she is on the best possible path. I assure you, that to this day I still have patients, a lot of them from America. Patients who have tumors in both breasts. I have the oils used externally as oil packs. I explain the diet as extensively as possible, everything that allopathy or natural medicin has worked out, whether cold water, thermal baths, or warm water, whether anthroposophy, pyschology is considered, horse hair mattresses are also very important.

Everything can be continue to used as well. But none of this will help at all if the person can no longer breathe. And the patients who come to me are numerous. Every week I receive hundreds of letters, I cannot answer all of them. I give my best, want to give my best, and I consider the engagement for this innovation, as a small part in of medicine in the turnaround of medicine as an obligation, which I accept before God and all people with total commitment and in all ernest. That is my contribution for this evening.

Presentation in Stuttgart

Assigned discussoin contribution on 24.09.98

Distinguished participants, I would like to start with a word of thanks to Mr. Wiewel, who has come here from the republic of scholars, these are people who realize science in harmony with the laws of nature. I was particularly impressed when all of you who were affected raised their hands. And I would like to assure you that the event this evening as the one held last night in Frankfurt, will comply with all the the rules listed by Mr. Wiewel. We only want to tell you the truth, and I obligate myself to do so.

And even if the basis of modern quantum physics seems baffling at first, I assure you that if you wil listen to me closely for the 10-15 minutes that are available to me, then you will know that the rainbow over cancer research, cancer therapy, and prevention is can be reached, and that it is a reality which all of you can use immediately. There were doctors who said, "I certainly can't prescribe flax oil if I don't know how flax oil works. I am of the opinion that no doctor can precisely anlyse how water works, and how it is that seeds grow in soil. To this day there is no doctor who can anlyse the effect of sun and water. However there are facts.

In the desert it is considered to be worse than murder if one who lives in the oasis, does not tell one who is thirsty where to find water. He who lives in the oasis, he who has water and sun available and rejoices in nature is obligated with the responsibility as a human being before God, to share this life giving substance, indeed with all people, so that they are awake and can realize this. It's right, you do not need to wait until that doctor, (this is certainly not the case with all of them), until that doctor who says. "I cannot prescribe flax oil", or who says; "I do not understand the rainbow, so I cannot use it, comes to your aid. If you think about it, you will realize that we are all a part of nature. The quantum physicist Werner Heisenberg has already demonstrated, I know him personally very well, that when representatives of old conceptual structures and the rigid old school want to force our new findings into their old conceptual structure, it simply does not work. We must be open. The clear findings of quantum physics, the interplay of electrons with soloar photons is fundamentally important for every life function.

The modest contribution that I have been able to make in this regard was that the highly unsaturated fatty acids, (for which there was were no verifications prior to my work), that these highly unsaturated fatty acids in their natural association are so rich in vital electrons, that they provide an incredible amount of energy in interaction with the sun. I proved this and indeed I proved it in government service in the State Health Office in the highest position responsible for pharmaceuticals and fats, 1952. In 1955 the Federal Ministry of Food wrote me to say that 6 international experts had confirmed my findings, and that the margarine industry had declared that they were prepared to change the way they processed oils.

He said that there would be no need for legislation. You can read in my book: Der Tod des Tumors Bd. II (The Death of the Tumor Vol. II). We are still waiting for this change in the industry, and what Mr. Frank Wiewel says is true, cancer patients are given false information in the press. I have given photocopies articles that appeared in yesterday's Schwarzwälder - Boten (local newspaper), to the organizers of this event, which announce that the pharmaceutical industry will now manufacture products for functional nutrition. They cannot do this. First it has long been demonstrated scientifically, that the vital photo elements stored in seed oils, recognized as vital in the fatty acids, cannot be produced in any industry to this day. And the same goes for vitamins.

The natural vitamins C, A, B, E are certainly important as vitamins. However they were not capable of regulating the reduced oxygen absorption in the respiratory enzymes. This was demonstrated through my work by adding the inserting the highly unsaturated fatty acids. In the meantime I have built on these findings and have developed my nutrition therapy.

When statements were published in Stockholm that there were other methods, I do not want to name them by name, there was again the difficulty of shelf life in the industry. When statements were published in New York, that said we couldn't treat cancer patients with lasers, because the burn damage is too extensive, that same year I oils which guided the absorption of the laser. By treating the patient in the lymph vessels and in the fat metabolism the tumors can be eliminated, even from the brain, this has been proven hundreds of times. If now a week ago someone from Heidelberg published that we have a new discovery to publicize, the use of laser beams against brain tumors, by boring just a small hole through the skullcap then the therapy built on this is untrue and dishonest and harmful to the patient.

Just using the nutrition therapy including the oils that are applied externally brings the tumor extensively to elimination because the normal growth processes apply this dynamic force also in the immune system of the human being. Naturally there is a limit, where the vital of function of the human being also fails. Often I am asked the question: "Is everything that we have learned as doctors useless?" – The answer is no! You can use hot water, cold water, homeopathy or psychology; all this is important, but everything is to no avail if a person's normal respiration is cut off by fats that have incorrectly been made to have a long shelf life, i.e. that hinder oxygen absorption. I do not want to go over my allotted time and advise you to have the courage to act for yourself. I am very grateful to the scientists who have come to us in Germany from the republic of scholars.

I am thankful for the new elite in science associated with truth who visit us here at this event and now encourage you to seek true help independently of those who only want to distribute water spoonful by spoonful, and make a business out of it. Do not lose sight of your right to life. There are enough people who stand up for truth. You who are sick and who are looking for help, avoid all the chaos and wrong that is out there. Go for natural help, it is near, like the dove that had an olive leaf in its beak, as it showed God's grace to the people in the rainbow. I wish you every success.

The following letter was requested by Frank Wiewel president of People against Cancer in response to an Internet report.

Biological cancer prevention through the growth powers of seed oils

"Successful non-conventional cancer therapies", this is how Frank Wiewel, president of People Against Cancer from the USA opened a series of presentations which audiences considered credible. The explanations were credible, that the chemotherapy we currently use is neither legitimate, nor scientific, nor has it been proven successful against metastases. The topic I have chosen was: "The rainbow over cancer research - cancer therapy and prevention".

It was clear that our book, which appeared in German and English: "KREBS - Das Problem und die Lösung ("CANCER – The Problem and the Solution) / Dr. Johanna Budwig: The Documentation", would be accepted. The other speakers also confirmed the significance of the fat issue for cancer therapy. The number of biological cancer therapies that are being offered is increasing, for example in a journal from Australia. What is widely publicized here is from David Horrobin The clinical uses of fatty acids and flax oil is given in capsules. Numerous patients from the USA come to me disappointed in "biological cancer therapy".

The core problem: I was successful as published in 1952, together with Professor Kaufmann, the director of the Federal Institute for Fats Research in producing the first verifications for fat and fatty acids using paper chromatography (see: Neue Wege der Fettanalyse, (New Directions in fat analysis)). 1950, in my activity at the State Health Office there were no methods to detect fats. 1952 we published jointly: Zur Biologie der Fette Die Papierchromatographie der Blutlipoide, Geschwulstproblem und Fettforschung." (On the Biology of Fats: paper chromatography of blood lipoids, ulcer problem and fat research."

I found out that the oxygen deficiency in living tissue is overcome through linoleic acid, ideally in conjunction with linolenic acid. According to Otto Warburg oxygen deficiency is considered to be the cause of cancer in the tumor-bearing tissue.

Thus I had found the 2nd pair in the autoxydable system of the cell, which had been sought for 100 years. Soon there followed our publication on "poly oils". The toxicity, which we had proven – also in the tumor-bearing tissue – has been confirmed by experts, as well as by the Federal Ministry of Food.

Every biological cancer therapy, which does not offer a clarification in this context, must fail. Flaxseed oil that is only administered in capsules cannot ensure a radical tumor therapy. Edible fats, made to have a long shelf life through industrial processes against oxygen absorption also disturb the autoxydable oxygen absorption in living tissue. Vitamin additives such as vit. A, B, C, D, and E do not provide any help if the respiratory enzymes are blocked by antioxidants. Vitamins follow their own laws for maintaining harmony among vitamins.

The misuse of the information concerning vitamin function as part of biological cancer therapies usually comes from those who exclude the core problem. Today every "biological cancer therapy" must also take the core problem into consideration. Man needs the vital powers, rich in electrons, that are built up in seeds from the energy of the sun and which direct all growth forces. Pseudo oils e.g. poly oils made to have a long shelf life disturb the healing process.

Cancer is a disease of the entire body. In therapy the entire life process must be given the possiblity to heal and to overcome the cancer disease.

The oil-protein diet that I have devloped is capable of breaking down and eliminating tumors and metastasis through the immune defence. To activate this process I also developed oils for external use – the ELDI oils. This was done as part of my inventive activity, to offer the electron systems of the fatty acids in flax oil, actively effective, in products that could be marketed.

My inventive activity was recognized by 3 ministers and was awarded the confirmation economically valuable. This expressly includes the making the products Linomel flaxseed and the ELDI oils preservable in a natural manner that maintains the electron systems that activate the respiratory function of cells – and that also are active in forming hemoglobin for hemopoieses (blood formation).

This privilige which had legally effective impact also includes treating paitents, "pioneering new ways in cancer research". This privilige clearly includes protection against those who are impacted by this inventive activity. Hostile growth inhibiting cancer therapies and edible fats which inhibit the respiratory function cause pain for the ill person. The ELDI oils (Electron Differentation oils) that I have produced cause the opposite. Pain institutes in the USA document: "What this woman accomplishes with her ELDI oils, none of us can accomplish using pain medication". A university appointed me to their scientific advisory board as an honorable member.

The activities of those affected in the rigid conceptual structures against the new of the inventive activity, must now be tested very carefully and conscientiously.

People in need notice and feel where truth rules.

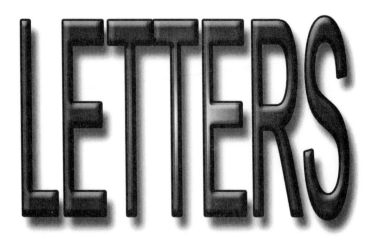

On the following pages you can read letters from my patients
that document the success of the oil-protein diet, but these
letters also demonstrate that professors, Deutsche Krebshilfe
(German Cancer Aid) and politicians have been aware of my
findings for decades.

In addition I refer to my book: Der Tod des Tumors, Band II
(The Death of the Tumor, Vol. II) which presents many
detailed reports from patients and physicians, some with
graphic material.

All of the original letters are at the publisher's without excep-
tion.

EUROPEAN Federation of Doctors

In German speaking countries e.V.

Associated with the

WORLD FEDERATION OF DOCTORS WHO RESPECT HUMAN LIFE

General Secretary: Ph.Schepens MD Derruyalaan, 76-B
8400 Ostend (Belgium)
Action office for the Federal Republic of Germany
PO box 1123, Römerstr. 20, 7900 Ulm/Danube
Telephone +49 731 / 3 04 49

1. Director Dr. Siegfried Ernst, Ulm
2. Director Dr. Georg Götz, Augsburg-Stadtbergen

To
Dr. Johanna Budwig
Freudenstadt-Dietersweiler

Re: Explanation of the submission to the financial authorities

Position on the treatment methods of Dr. Budwig.

I had an operation on the 21st of March 1978, performed by Professor Christian Herfarth (he is now head surgeon of the Surgery Clinic of the University of Heidelberg) because of a large stomach carcinoma which had already grown through to the large intestine, and which was on the external limit of operability. Because I rejected after-care with cytostatic agents, after a detailed discussion with Dr. Johanna Budwig, I decided to undergo her treatment with the oil-protein diet and application of ELDI oils.

This resulted in a constant progressive gradual improvement of the general condition, particularly also in the entire immune situatiuon of the organism against virus infections etc. A follow-up examination in July 1983 at the Ulm University Clinic department of internal medicine by Dr. Pfeiffer produced no indications whatsoever for a carcinomatosis event, so that now after 5 ½ years the carcinoma can be considered to be healed-up.

It is my medical and scientific conviction that changing the diet to Dr. Budwig's oil-protein diet and the corresponding treatment with the ELDI oils played a significant role.

Dr. med. Siegfried Ernst

Graduate Engineer
Fritz Kirchner
Lilienstr. 25

66 Saarbrücken 1

27.5.1983

INTER Krankenversicherung AG.
Saaruferstr.14

6600 Saarbrücken 1

Re: Policy. no.:
        Medical treatment of my wife Maria Kirchner

Dear Sir or Madam,

In the fall of 1982, in the lymph node examination of my
wife, metastases were detected. Subsequent examinations
detected additional metastases along the breast milk duct, as
well as on the fallopian tube. I was told that my wife could
not be cured. I was informed that through treatment with
cytostatic agents the physicians could only slow the progres-
sion of the disease, however this treatment would involve
considerable side effects.

My wife and I refused this treatment.

In the search for alternative cancer treatment methods I found the therapy according to Dr. Budwig. A women from Saarlouis, who suffered from a sarcoma was treated in this manner, and after 10 years she has no medical disorders.

Now since January 1983 my wife has also been successfully treated by Dr. Budwig.

Supported by the court decision that the cancer patient is also entitled to look to alternative methods for healing, and that the insurance company must bear the costs, I submit to you the enclosed listing of the expenses incurred thus far. I request that the sum of DM ... be reimbursed to me within 6 weeks. I hope that we can avoid a legal dispute, particularly as my wife who was seriously ill has been doing very well since the therapy with Dr. Budwig.

Regards,

Fritz Kirchner

Jürg Hülf
Husumerstr. 7

2000 Hamburg 20

To the
Allgemeine Ortskrankenkasse Hamburg
Kaiser-Wilhelm-Str. 93

2000 Hamburg 36

Hamburg, July 11th 1993

Dear Sir or Madam,

According to your documents, in September 1980 I was diagnosed with an adenoid, cystic carcinoma of the tear duct in the left orbital area.

In spite of an extensive operation and removal of the left eyeball, since september 1982 there has been a relapse. This was then removed, as it was the first time, by Dr. M. in the department of oral and maxillofacial surgery in the Oschsenzoll hospital.

There was a risk of the carcinoma spreading and encroaching on the remaining eye.

In light of this situation I decided to use the well-proven treatment method of Dr. Johanna Budwig. This method is scientifically substantiated, published in medical journals, and is presented at congresses in Germany and abroad.

Personally I have only benefitted from using the oil-protein diet and the Eldi oils.

a) The wound healed in an astonishingly short time.

b) Vision in the remaining eye improved, I wear glasses, by more than one dioptrine from 5.8 previosly to the present – 4.6.

c) In the the forehead area, after the first operation hair fell out in the receding hairline area. Now hair has grown back in this area.

d) My blood pressure normalized in a short time and is currently optimal.

e) I was able to resume my work after a short time. I feel very good in body and in spirit.

f) The frequent migraine headaches experienced prior to the second operation rarely occur and they can be handled without medication.

g) A tooth infection which caused extreme pain healed in a short time without dental care.

h) Because my family also strictly follows the oil-protein diet, my wife's chronic constipation disappeared and so did her vegetative dystonia, which was treated by doctors for years without success. Similar experiences can also be reported for my children.

Such a treatment result would not have been possible without the contiuing personal engagement of Dr. Budwig.

I hereby request compensation for the costs incurred through this treatment.

According to the recently clarified legal position I expect payment to my bank account for the costs listed in the attachment by the 15th of August 1983.

Regards,

Jörg Hulf

Attachments
Itemized costs
Receipts for the individual cost types

Westphalia

Dear Dr. Budwig,

I am happy to comply with your request and make my case history available to you to use as you please. In early 1993 I noticed a small lump on the right side of the tip of my tongue. Because my doctor assured me that it was completely harmless, and because it really irritated me I had it removed in the ear, nose and throat clinic by Professor A. Even during the operation I noticed that there was something wrong. That evening my tongue had swollen to three times its normal size and was almost black. I had severe pain and had to stay in the clinic for three days due to the danger of secondary hemorrhage. In the clinic I was expressly assured that the lump was completely harmless.

After about a week the hospital told me on the phone that I had salivary gland cancer. In a subsequent discussion I learned that the Professor had had major difficulties with the operation. The lump was not delimited; rather the cancer had already spread in the tongue. A new operation was prescribed without asking me for my consent. This time with general anesthesia because this operation would involve a greater scope than the first. I refused and returned home totally shocked.

I called Dr. Budwig who had already helped me wonderfully years before, and an appointment was arranged for the following week. After this meeting I was very collected and in good spirits. In the meantime I got a call from our family doctor at the time who requested that I come to his practice for a talk. With the assumption that he wanted to encourage me and that he would support me in my decision, I went to him. Without any human emotion he brutally explained to me that only an operation (removal of ¾ of the tongue) could save me, if at all. Then he listed everything in great detail that would not help me, and how the cancer would continue to spread in my body over time.

At the same time he wanted me to meet a patient who had had her tongue removed recently, and who was doing very well. He would not allow me to speak. He said that this would be the only possibility that could still help me (at least for a short time). Thereafter naturally the doctors would be powerless, as this type of cancer was totally incurable. An operation however would somewhat prolong the situation.

I refused the operation. Then he forgot all good manners and he was very abusive. He berated me, he said that I would never survive if I did not go into the clinic immediately for an operation. I said no, to which he bellowed: OK die then, no God, no prayer can help you. During this entire time he did not offer me a single word of encouragement. I left the practice totally distraught. All hope of healing was gone. This doctor literally pulled the rug out from under my feet. This bordered on psycho-terror. Totally crushed my husband drove me to Dr. Budwig. She calmed me and she gave me new hope through her special and unique manner and spirit.

At home I immediately started with the oil-protein diet from Dr. Budwig, after precise instructions. I could call whenever I needed a talk and support. After a few days, however the discussion with the family doctor really got to me again. His threats kept going through my head and soon I could not think of anything else. I had terrible nightmares; soon I had them every night. My husband was barely able to calm me after such a dream. My fear grew to immeasurable proportions. In the dream I always died under the worst conditions imaginable. Soon I could no longer be alone because of my fear. I lost interest in everything; it was hard to eat anything. I always thought, "It's just not worth it anymore I will die soon anyway". These were the two worst years of my life. This doctor had simply sentenced me to death and I was not capable of freeing myself from this vicious circle.

I can no longer recall how often I telephoned with Dr. Budwig or saw her in Dietersweiler. The fear handicapped me completely. I believe I could neither communicate to my family nor to Dr. Budwig the miserable condition I was caught in. When I spoke with Dr. Budwig, I felt better, but after a short time the old condition returned. But with the true patience of an angel, with never failing understanding, she helped me through this worst of times.

If I had died at that time, (for a long time I was thoroughly convinced that this would be the case), then it would not have been due to my cancer illness, (I was in the best of hands), but rather it would have been due to the irresponsibility of this doctor. After two years of indefatigable encouragement on the part of Dr. Budwig, and the fact that I was still alive, the nightmares became less frequent and the panic-like anxiety slowly dissipated entirely. I was no longer full of panic, and I no longer turned around and walked in the other direction if I chanced to encounter this doctor.

I forced myself to walk by him very calmly. And suddenly I noticed that he avoided me (it was probably awkward for him that nothing that he had threatened me with had occurred). I survived the illness thanks to Dr. Budwig. Today I am again a happy and balanced individual. The oil-protein diet tastes wonderful to me (and to my husband) and I strictly observe all guidelines. I am full of gratitude that God directed me to Dr. Budwig. How terrible a life without a tongue would have been, if I had survived at all.

Please contact Dr. Budwig if there are questions concerning my case.

A. Sch.
(Westphalia)

Dr. G. A. Skoupka
Hartenfelsweg 5

5000 Cologne

30.07.1983

Dear Dr. Budwig,

Now that 5 weeks have passed, since I agreed with you for the first time, I would like to send you a brief summary report of the course of my husbund's illness.

After my husbund suffered for months with major disorders (coughing, spitting up blood, labored breathing) he suffered an acute choking fit on the 9th of June 1983. He was taken immediately to the emergency room at the Univesity Clinik in Cologne where he was diagnosed with a bronchial carcinoma. The doctors considered my husbund's life-expectancy to be very limited with irradiation and chemotherapy.

At this time (June 17th 1983) I turned to you for help. On your advice I took my husbund out of the hospital on the following day. His condition at this time was still poor (strong coughing, spitting up blood, labored breathing). We started immediately with the oil-protein diet and external treatment with ELDI oils. He immediately stopped taking all medications that had been prescribed in the hospital (more than a dozen).

My husbund's condition improved noticiably immediately. The labored breathing that my husbund suffered up to his last day in the hospital, disappeared completely. In the 5 weeks of the oil-protein diet he has been getting stronger and stronger, the disease characteristics are giving way to a condition that is almost completely normal.

Best regards and with sincere thanks

Dorothea Skorupka

Werner Schwarz
Federal Minister of Food, Agriculture and Forestry

05. October 1961

To the
Federal Minister of the Interior
Dr. Gerhard Schröder

Bonn

Dear Colleague

I refer to a letter written to you by Dr. Johanna Budwig from Bad Zwischenau dated September 26th this year, and of which I have received a copy. I know Dr. Budwig, as several years ago she gave a presentation to the agriculture work group of our faction on the problems of proper nutrition and thus cancer prevention, which very much impressed all of us at that time.

Naturally I cannot evaluate Dr. Budwig's medical theories and views. Nevertheless I am of the opinion that such a serious issue as fighting ancer is justification enough to leave nothing untried, and if necessary to devote resources to support research that deviates from views that have been previously represented. Consequently I would be very pleased if you could find a way to accommodate the request of Dr. Budwig.

I would appreciate a brief message as to whether, and possibly in which manner, help can be provided in this regard.

Regards,

Werner Schwarz

To Ms.
Dr. Johanna Budwig
Helgelstr. 3

D - 72250 Freudenstadt (Dietersweiler)

Wädenswil 28.07.1999

Dear Dr. Budwig,

I am pleased to report my current condition to you, approximately 10 years after my first consultation with you.

The condition of my affected right eye which at that time was worsening week-by-week stabilised in a positive sense shortly after starting treatment in accordance with your advice. The CT findings at that time showed an optic nerve, which had thickend by more than 30% with a differential diagnosis evaluation of glioma, neurinoma or meningioma. An operation was advised and was scheduled to take place shortly thereafter.

I can use the affected eye as a functional organ, which was previously the case. A certain loss as residual condition has remained, but there is no trace of the illness that I had at that time. Since I have been following the counsel you gave me, I feel significantly more capable, I can handle what needs to be handled and I do not need a doctor. By the way I no longer go in for medical exams or treatment.

You will understand my joy and I am very grateful to you for the counsel you have given me.

With all my heart I wish you all the best.

Regards,

R.I.
CH –

Johann Barend Krebs
428 East 11th Street
North Vancouver BC

Canada, V7L 2H2

July 8th 1999

Dear Dr. Budwig,

I have some very good news for you. What I had felt for a long time and basically knew for myself has now been confirmed by my physician, Dr. Florence Yakura MD in Burnaby, BC and by the opthamalogist Dr. James Thompson. No tumor can be detected any more, and the optic nerve on which the tumor had exerted pressure has regenerated itself. In addition, my vital energy has returned and at age 55 I feel 20 years younger. This brought us great joy and we express our gratitude to the creator of life and particularly to you. We greatly admire your work and courage in going your own way against the existing and established medical model. Personally I very grateful to you.

Friends, acquaintances, colleagues at the university where I work often comment on how healthy I look, and when they hear my story, they often say that it is miracle that I am so healthy again. Then I say, it is not a miracle, it is pure biology. It is a miracle that I heard about Dr. Budwig (through

German friends) who is one of the few people in the world who understands the factors in the body that play a role in cancer and turmors and their treatment.

As you will remember I had a pituitary tumor (adenoma) and I was operated on for the first time in 1982. In 1993 the tumor was again diagnosed and since that time I have been looking for a natural method of treating the tumor. Because the tumor was still small, I had some time, however I postponed having an operation, in order to try out other methods. In December 1996 I could no longer see the color red and should have had an operation. But I was only ready for an operation at the end of August, because I couldn't wait any longer, and also I had no other prospect for a natural cure. My doctor showed me regularly what the condition was and told me clearly that I could not afford to wait any longer. I had already waited long enough. I could barely see. In spite of this I decided to postpone the operation once again, tried another promising therapy but the tumor did not dissolve, and then when I heard about you I went to see you in October 1997. I spent four days with you and learned what to do. Two weeks later I started to feel better, three weeks later I felt how my facial capacity was beginning to improve, and six months later I had the feeling that the tumor was probably gone. Now this has been confirmed from the medical side. Thank you again. May God bless you.

With much warmth and esteem

Johann Barend Krebs

Brkki Halme

Dear Dr. Augstein!

It was nice to get your letter 25.11.83. You have done work of great merits when working so many years of Dr. Budwig´s lawyer. I am also affirmed that Dr. Budwig is one scientist of the most of genius in the whole world, good comparabel with Einstein, Max Planck, Louis Broglie, Niels Bohr or as well Ignas Semmelweis.

Dr. Budwigs work is extremly important for the cancer research and it is also important of the cure of cancer. The orthodoxy medical-scientists cure cancer after 5 years in 16 % and Dr. Budwig cures it in 90 %.

There is a good example abouth faith in authority that is not willingly to acknowledge absolutely simple truths. Also Nobel-committees supports obviously this kind of faith in authority. The committee whose 50 members are professors of Karolinska institute is mainly made up of representatives of orthodox medicine, and they have difficult to comprehend that only the Budwigs natural course of action and after its ground working acts are the unique method in recovering from cancer. I will try once more for Nobel price.

Sincerely

Prof. Brkke Halme

Min.-Rat Dr. Hensen in Federal Ministry
of Food, Agriculture and Forestry"

III B 4- 3833.24-376/54

Bonn, 25th of June 1955

Dr. Budwig
Münster/Westf.
Wienerstr. 33

Regarding polymerized fish oil.

Dear Dr. Budwig,

In July 1951 I commissioned the Institute for Virus Research
and Experimental Medicine in Sielbeck bei Eutin, to test the
usability of polymerised fats for human consumption. The
institute's report was suitable, to act with maximum caution
relative to polymerized oils for the human diet. Further
experiments which I had performed by the German Institute
for Fats Research in Münster reinforced this impression and
induced me to advise utmost reserve in the use of polymerized fats, to the German fish industry, as well as to the
German margarine industy. After submission of the test
results, jointly with the Fenderal Minister of the Interior, I
have considerd a ban on products that are manufactured
using polymerized oils. Because such a ban could only be

limited to the German interior, in September 1953 there was a discussion with scientists from Norway, as Norway was very interested in the export of industrial fish products using polymerized oils. The following people participated in this discussion:

From the Norwegian side:
Prof. Dr. R. Nikolaysen, Oslo, University institute for nutritional research,
Prof. Dr. 0. Togersen, Oslo, University Institute for pathology, Rikshospitalet,
Dr. ing. chem. H. Nilsen-Moe, Oslo, Hermetics laboratory, Stavanger,

On the German side:
Prof. Dr. Kärber, Berlin-Dahlem, Max von Pettenkofer Institute German Federal Health Office,
Prof. Dr. Dr. K. Lang, Mainz, Physiol-chem. Institute at the University,
Dr. H. Frahm, Kiel, Waigmannstr., Bact. Institut der Federal Dairy Farming Research Institute,
Dr. H. Werner, Hamburg, Chemical and Foodstuffs Testing Center of the Publich Health Authority.

In the discussion the Norwegian experts could not dispel the concerns put forward by the German side. Although requested repeatedly the Norwegian side did not send samples of the Norwegian oils used. The Federal Research Center for Fisheries in Hamburg, determined that the imported canned fish now coming in no longer contains polymerized oils.

The Chair of the Federal Health Office communicated to me in December last year that since the Hamburg discussion on the 8th of September 1953 that there no longer seems to be any special interest in the polymerized oil issue.

Thus the health damage, associated with consumption of polymerized oils, that you have feared, has also been confirmed from another scientific side, and through the development that has now ensued in the meantime, is considered to be resolved. I thank you for the help that you provided in this issue.

I have sent a copy of this letter to the Dr. Hedwig Jochmus, Member of the Bundestag (German Parliament).

With best regards

respecfully

signed Dr. H. Hensen.

Dr. Mittmann
Cancer Research
North Rhine-Westphalia
Statistical Department
(22c) Bonn-Venusberg
Skin Clinic
25. 9. 57

Prof. Dr. L. Erhard,
Federal Minister of Economy
Bonn-Venusberg
Schleichstr. 8

Regarding: Aftermath to correspondence dated 14 September 1957

Dear Minister!

The two reprints with accompanying letter dated September 14th 1957 represent two publications of a publication series of 3 works, the third work is currently being printed. As it will be some time before the third work will appear, by your leave I send you a manuscript copy.

The results obtained through statistical methods of my publication series harmonize with results of other researchers who do not work statistically, particularly O. WARBURG and J. BUDWIG. I was referred to Ms. Budwig, who comes from the chemistry side, by Professor H. MARTIUS (Göttingen) although in his capacity as president of the German Central Committee for the Prevention of Cancer and Cancer Research, officially he cannot take a positive position to BUDWIG's results. By the way the BUDWIG results have now been confirmed by NYROP (Copenhagen) and SIN-CLAIR (Oxford).

With best regards

respecfully
signed Mittmann

Fritz Zeller
Münsterplatz 45

79 Ulm-Donau

To the Ministery of Health
To Minister Antje Huber

24.01.1981

Dear Minister!

Yesterday, June 23rd,1981 an article appeared in the Südwest Presse with the headline: "Little success in the fight against cancer". This article said that in the first session of the Bundestag this year you explained in the cancer report: "We can't refer to a real improvement in the area of research – a breakthrough in the fight against cancer is not yet in sight. Unfortunately that is the truth and annually 150,000 people die of cancer in Germany according to the statistics.
Please take my case into consideration:

I have myself examined for cancer at least once a year and and the result is always: "no findings". But to be sure at the end of 1979 I consulted a university professor, the success was that a prostate operation was performed immediately on me in the university clinic, and a cancerous tumor in the prostate was removed.

In a subsequent second operation the testes were also removed and a bone scintigram was performed with the result: "Multple metastases in the entire axial skeleton".

After these operations and examinations the treating doctor had my wife come to him because he did not want to tell me the truth due to my poor condition, and he told her that I could no longer be helped and that I had to consider a maximum life expectency of two years.

Then by chance after I was released from the hospital I came to be treated by a biologist, a homeopathic practitioner, who prior to treating me had already helped hundreds of cancer patients who had been given up on by doctors as incurable. Through the strict diet that she prescribed I started feeling better right from the start and now after two years, I had a second scintigram performed at the same university, and wonder of wonders – the results had so improved that metastases could no longer be determined with certainty.

Recently I brought this healing method to the attention of the Deutsche Krebshile (German Cancer Aid) and requested that they research these extraordinary successes. After some time I got a response from the Deustsche Krebshilfe (German Cancer Aid) that "in funding research projects, only those projects will be funded that cannot elude scientific verification". To this I say:

The entire area of cancer research moves in well-traveled paths and in living memory this has always been the case, that established findings and principles of science are defended with all resources against people with other ideas, who consider these findings and principles to be incorrect, and that outsiders are fought.

I, and many other fellow sufferers thank this scientist for the healing. In decades of research, in the frontier area of biology, chemistry, physics, and medicine this scientist traced the causes of cancer and came to the conclusion that cancer is a fat problem, and that it can be treated successfully by changing the diet. Her findings are very uncomfortable for allopathy and consequently she is fought by many medical practitioners and also by the margarine union; the intent is to muzzle this researcher with at all costs.

I request that you pursue the information in my report, and after careful review of the documents help yourself to a breakthrough in the fight against cancer. The name and address of the researcher:

Dr. Johanna Budwig, 72550 Dietersweiler-Freudenstadt, Tel: 07441-7667 Fax: 07441-85125

She holds a doctorate from the philosophic and natural science faculties, and state examinations, in physics and pharmacy.

I would be very happy to see that other paths of cancer fighting are also pursued through her initiative.

Respectfully,

Fritz Zeller

City of Stuttgart
Katharinen Hospital Radiology Clinic
Medical director: Dr. med. W. Hellriegel

Ms.

Dr. Johanna Budwig

7291 Lauterbad
über Freudenstadt

Dear Dr. Budwig,

Recently you treated one of my patients, Ms. Harriet ------, born on December 4th 1931. With this patient there was a malignant melanoma on the left femur, which was surgically removed in May 1969 in Ohio .

In September 1970 there was a lymph node metastasis on the left temple, which degenerated after radiation treatment, also the subsequent lymph node metastases in January 1971 on the left side of the throat were brought to degeneration through radition treatment. In March 1971 there was general worsening as there was a generalised metastasis in the skin. Multiple skin metastases could be detected on the torso.

After treatment with you all lymph node and skin metastases have degenerated. Moreover all blood chemistry findings have normalized. I have never observed such a result in the case of metastatizing malignant melanomas. I would be extermely grateful if you would tell me which therapy you performed.

As I currently have other patients with the same illness and the same poor condition, I would be happy to send these patients to you to delay the recognizable end of these patients.

On the other hand, Naturally I am also prepared to use this therapy here if you would communicate this method to me.

I would be very pleased to get a message from you. Until then

Regards,

Your

Dr. med. W. Hellriegel

Klaus Hiller
Senior Criminal Director
Kaiserstr. 6

77963 Schwanau

27.09.1997

Dear Dr. Budwig,

Your 90th birthday is an occoasion for my spouse and me to congratulate you most sincerely and wish you continued good health, but it is also an occasion to thank you once again for your magnificent efforts in the healing of my spouse.

You will certainly recall the state of my spouse when we sought your help more than 13 years ago.

Due to a laryngeal carcinoma the entire larynx had been removed. In this operation metastases were detected in the lymph nodes and thyroid gland. What was particularly alarming was the degree to which the metastases had spread, which at the time had already infiltrated the surrounding soft tissue and were already necrotic.

The treating physician at the Erlangen Clinic, Dr. Steiner represented the opinion at that time that even with subsequent radiation treatment, which he considered to indispensible, my wife's life expectency would not be significantly longer than about 1 year.

Details from the disease pattern are documented in the enclosed attachment.

We decided for the biological therapy that you developed and did not pursue radiation treatment and stopped any further medical treatment. This decision saved my spouse finally from that death that had appeared to be certain. We thank you for this.

In conclusion I would like to mention again that we have moved from Stuttgatt to the Freiburg area. My new address is on the letterhead; the new tel. number is ------. I am also enclosing a card with my office address address.

All the best

Your

Klaus Hiller

University Erlangen-Nürnberg

Clinic and Polyclinic for ear nose and throat patients

Dr. med. Hans Melchior Hofmeier
Ear nose and throat physician
Paracelsusweg 9

7302 Ostfildern 1 Ruit

20.05.1985

Dear Colleague

Here is a summary report concerning our common patient Ms. Sonja Hiller who received in-patient treatment from March 25th 1985 to March 29th 1985, as well as from April 24th 1985 to May 15th 1985.

Please permit me to make some preliminary comments on the prehistory, which I have essentially taken from your letter dated March 14th 1985, supplemented by the patient's own information, because I am of the opinion that the disease pattern and the course of the illness are quite unusual.

According to the patient's own information, the young

patient, a non-smoker, had been suffering from a voice disorder for approximately 2 years. In early 1984 she underwent voice and speech therapy at the Katharinen Hospital in Stuttgart. In August 1984 the patient first sought your help due to hoarseness and labored breathing. Layngealscopically they found a full-blown subglottal edema at a width of the subglottis of 2-3 mm, vocal cords and vocal cords could not be stimulated, the right vocal cord lagged behind somewhat during phonation. In the assumption that there was relationship with the known allergy to house dust and the present pregnancy (month 5), at first she underwent a conservative treatment and sought a change of climate.

However, after a transitory improvement, worsening again occurred in October 1984, which is why she underwent a conservative treatment under in-patient conditions. Then after delivery of the child through C-section in December 1984, you again treated the patient consertivaly with cortisone and other medications. However since no essential improvement occurred you executed a microlaryngoscopy under anesthesia on May 3rd 1985.

Do to a significant subglottal stenosis the intubations was difficult, the vocal fold function was intact. In the glottal area to the right of the front commisure starting and extending to the larynx area you removed the granulations, which then, in a histologically surprising manner, showed a non-squamous cell epithelial carcinoma. The patient was then referred to Professor Kittel, the director of the Erlanger Voice and Speech department, who entrusted me with the further care of the patient.

Endoscopically the patient had granulating changes mainly in the right dorsal subglottal area however without clinically certain signs of malignancy. With consideration of the clinical histological discrepancy I first performed a microlaryngoscopic diagnostic laser excision under intubation for general anesthesia on March 27th 1985. Because the frozen section examination of an excision biopsy in the area right rear vocal fold area resulted in a carcinoma in situ, I immediately carried out a post-resection in the same intervention. The treatment of this specimen then revealed a micro carcinoma.

A concluding epicritical histological synopsis performed by Professor Pesch in the Erlanger Pathological Institute from the preparations kindly provided by Professor Schneider in Esslingen, together with the excisions which we had obtained revealed, according to the letter dated April 4th 1985, that there was no doubt as to the malignancy of the clinically non-suspicious proliferations, an invasively growing, moderately differentiated squamous cell epithelial carcinoma was present. It is highly probable that the operation was not performed in healthy tissue, because there was urgent suspicion of a lymphogenic metastasis.

In consideration of this finding, in order to be certain, a microlaryngeal laser post-resection was performed in the right dorsal larynx, in spite of the clinically satisfying aspect of the endolarynx. The frozen section examination revealed that the entire excision was riddled by tumor; after consultation with family members I performed a laryngofissure, in the same session. In the attempt to retain functional important larynx structures for the young woman through a bilateral vertical partial resection, for a definitive rehabilitation, I applied an epithelized laryngotracheostoma; at the same time I performed an explorative regional functional neck dissection on the right side. Because intraoperative, histologically assured, the urgent suspicion of a very extended growing submucosal carcinoma was revealed, which had broken through prelaryngeally in the area of the front commissure, and cricoid cartilage and trachea had been afflicted, I decided on very extensive bilateral resections which affected thyroid cartilage, and cricoid cartilage as well as trachea, still in the same session.

The final treatment of the numerous post-resections and perimeter samples unfortunately now revealed histologically such an extended affection of thyroid cartilage, cricoid cartilage, and trachea with precricoidal breakthrough, as well as a lymphangiosis carcinomatosa and a caudal and lateral lymph node metastasis of the perivascular sheath, that a laryngectomy could not be avoided. On the 3rd of May 1985 I performed the intervention, in this process simultaneously a regional functional neck dissection was performed left and the regional neck clearance right was extended, skin tracheal portions were generously post-resected, in this process a lymph node metastasis was removed both paratracheal right which was more pronounced than left, which was localized between thyroid gland and trachea.

The right relatively large metastasis was necrotic; histologically there was an infiltration of the surrounding soft tissue. The right thyroid gland was removed completely; left portions of the thyroid gland were retained as only a small lymph node had been detected.

The atypical incision on the neck is due to the preliminary attempt at a larynx resection. The postoperative development had no complications. On the May 10th 1985, thus on the 8th postoperative day, the stomach probe could be removed. Considering the advanced larynx carcinoma (pT4) with affection of the thyroid cartilage and extra-laryngeal spreading with the caudal extension in the cricoid and the trachea, with the bilateral (pN3) metastasis, with capsule rupture right, post operative irradiation of both sides of the neck with mediastinum is urgently indexed. While the family members were instructed about the absolute oncological necessity of this irradiation therapy, the patient after speaking with the family members only knows about a post-operative irradiation, just to be sure, without having being told about the throat metastasis.

Because the patient had lived for at least 1 year with her parents-in-law in the vicinity of Freiburg, I requested that the patient undergoe the radiation therapy at the radiology clinik where Professor Wannenmacher is the director, and also have the after-care examinations as well as the esophagal speech therapy carried out in the ear nose & throat clinic where Professor Beck is the director. A primary surgical rehabilitiation of the voice after laryngectomy unfortunately was not possible due to the extended tumor resection. If the patient should have difficulties with learning esophagal method of speaking then a secondary prosthetic accommodation could be considered. I would be grateful if a distant metastases search and a possible immunological examination could be organized by the clinics in Freiburg. I thank you for the friendly handling of the further diagnosis and therapy of the young, patient who has been dealt with severly by fate.

With the best collegial regards

Dr. med. W. Steiner
Head physician of the clinic

Dr. Johanna Budwig

My most important scientific discoveries and the insights that can be based on them.

New facts and conclusions

1. My ideas in 1949: It must certainly be possible to produce verifications for chemistry of fats. Boldingh questioned this in writing. I was successful with these sensitive and specfic fat chemistry verifications.

2. The long desired, yes necessary, differential reaction e.g. between oil acid and linoleic acid was successful.

3. The paper chromotography of fats that Ideveloped with Professor Kaufmann (1949; 1950; 1951) spread tempestuously and world wide through publications at congresses, in the journal "Oil & Soap", also together with several professors and doctoral students, through which this method was extended. I developed control of the atmosheres in the closed system by using gas systems which act as antioxidants. Coloring, separating effects of fats and fatty acids were further developed. Behavior was studied in blue light, red light, with floursescent dyes. I noticed for example the electrical behavior of the unsaturated fatty acids with their "halo" using dyes with rhodamine red.

4. The impetus to immediately start the examination of blood fats was provided for example by the work by Nonnenbruch; the missing verifications for blood fats has a sensitive effect in medicine (1951).

5. Use of paper chromotography, Examination of Blood lipoids (published in 1952) immediately caused a furor. The cancer problem was brought in. The fats which were made preservable chemically, which includes all trans-fatty acids proved to be inhibiting substances in the metabolism of solids.

6. The resistance which had continued in the year prior to publication of the above-mentioned study (March 1952) allowed me to perform very thorough work to substantiate the importance of these findings.

7. It was proved, as I had published:

a) The linoleic acid or flax oil acids supply the second pair in the autoxydable system of the living cell, which had been sought by a specialized branch of science.

b) The inclusion of the physical chemistry of B. Eistert supplied me with immediately enlightening findings on the syngergism of the sulfhydryl group of protein with the Pi electrons of the highly unsaturaged fatty acids and their significance for the formation of lipopoteides, of the hydrogen bridge between fat and protein, which represent the only path for fast and focused transport of electrons in biological systems. On this basis the use of laser radiation for cancer patients succeeded for the first time.

c) This electron, built up of photons of sunlight e.g. in the photosynthesis in plants, also shows – on the threshold between light and matter – in the electon systems of the movable electron clouds that can be detached from matter, the Pi electrons of the highly unsaturaged fatty acids, the resonance capacity for the sun, which the human organism needs for its vital function: Respiration, growth, cell division, nerve function, secretions, build-up and breakdown of cells. There is no animal whose brain function is so highly capable, and so dependent on the absorbtion, storage, and reactivation of solar energy as is man (see "Photo effect" according to Einstein and the physics of realitivity). All vital functions of man are affected by this. The turning point in the field of cancer research and the proven successful cancer therapy are only one aspect of much bigger picture.

Findings in theoretical physics:

1. In 1900, Max Planck recognized the "Planck's constant", the universally applicable natural constant as quant of all radiation, of heat and black radiation.

2. Albert Einstein recognized and proved the quantum theory of light: The photon, quanta of light, is always accompanied by electromagnetic fields. The field is crucial for all exchanges of energy. Einstein proved with the photo effect: When irradiating a metal plate, for example, there is an exchange of energy in accordance with the frequency of the incoming energy, i.e. in accordance with the quality, not the quantity of the radiation. According to this quantum theory of light, space and time are drawn into the relativity, however electrical charge and entropy are not.

3. In 1924, Prince Louis de Broglie mathematically proved the radiation capacity of all matter, the matter waves, the duality of the light photon, always corpuscle, matter and at the same time the purest wave. He successfully applied this complementarity, the two faces of the photon to the electron and thus created quantum mechanics.

4. Niels Bohr had described the complementarity of the electron in hydrogen, with its volatile, quantum change of the energy level.

5. K.W. Ford, nuclear physisct, provides a fascinating description of the outstanding role accorded to the photon of sunlight, wherein the electron is a not a "completely lifeless object." The state of the great order "with color and inner activity", the leitmotif that also rules our world, from the theory of relativity (Einstein) to quantum mechanics (Louis de Broglie), and for the world of elementary particles substantiated by K. Ford. These three researchers also and emphasized this state in conjunction with the creation, as it maintains order through the "gentle substance of the wave fields"over the chaos of a probability.

6. Only the radiation of the artificial radioisotopes (K. Ford) with their positions is able to neutralize photons and electrons in their charge. This promotes entropy and death.

7. Friedrich Dessauer oberved in studies on radiation, described in "Quantum Biology" how important the "right rays" are for the energy depot for man. The role of the "big molecule" remained important to him but unknown.

My own findings:

The wonderful role of the photon of solar energy, also incorporated for us in food, gives us the resonance absorbtion for the solar energy. The gentle wave fields of the photons are indespensible for all energy exchange in the vital function of man. The change between light and matter in photons and to the accordant electrons is a core component in the vital function of human beings for all energy reserve and adaptation in accordance with the laws of relativity. It is also a core component in preventing illness.

Here hydrogen as the lightest atom, between energy and matter, in the hydrogen bridge, in the lipoproteides, bridge between fat and protein, plays crucial role as antie-entropy factor, as life promoting, the capability of hydroben to absorb quantum energy, conduct it and release it, is important in this process.

The radiations used in offocial allopathic medicine, with synthetically produced radioiosotopes works against this life process. It breaks down existing energy depots, destroys the gentle substance of the magnetic fields (spin of the electrons) which are indespensible for the energy transport in human beings.

I have been able to demonstrate in practice now for 20 years the extent to which the damage done to cancer patients who had been treated with irradiation, and who were totally reduced in the vital function, can be restored by supplying the necessary solar electron systems.

Where the quanta rule in accordance with the ultra-light photon, where the pilot wave is ruled by the duality wave/corpuscle of sunlight, that is also where for cancer patients, the initiated chaos is overcome. The control elements for the vital function of man in his individuality are supplied in the wave field of solar energy.

Important foundations for the theoretical physics and its biological quantum biology were provided by the books:

K.W. Ford: The World of Elementary Particles.

T. Thunberg: The Biological Significance of the Sulfhydryl Group (1911) and the treatment by Torsten Thunberg in the manual from B. Flaschenträger vol. 1 (1951).

I. Bang: Chemistry and Biochemistry of Lipoids (1911).

O. Warburg: On the Metabolism of Tumors (1926)

Louis de Broglie: Light and Matter (1949)
                    Physics and Microphysics (1950)

A. Einstein: Quantum law of Emission and Absorbtion of light, and on the meaning of the field in the movement of light

Fr. Dessauer: Quantum Biologie Issue 1954

Essential fatty acids in the vital function of the human organism

Introduction: On the state of tumor therapy.

If one precisely examines the occurrence of cancer, then there are indications that a relationship must exisit with our food. But definite starting points that could be helpful in proceeding against cancer have rarely been offered.

However the increasing efforts to get aid using propaganda in order to be successful in the fight against cancer, and the rapid increase in the incidence rate of these diseases are definite facts. The list of carcinogenic substances grows from year to year. The search for a general cancer therapy has lead to an erroneous trend, this situation has continued to this day. It is a proven fact in the establishment, that the goal of all cancer therapy is to stop the growth of cells. It is an essential factor in all carcinogenesis and in the failure of all cancer therapy, that the human organism fails in adaptation. In the following remarks a new point is now shown where the point of attack against cancer is successful.

I summarize how I substantiate the new ideas for a successful cancer therapy, which represents the absolute opposite of everything that has been previously attempted. It is my goal to promote the growth processes, particularly with the cancer cells.

The highly unsaturaged fatty acids will now be shown as substances, which through their activity, accelerate the growth rate of cell division - also the division cancer cells, and thus self-destruction of the tumor. De-differention of the cells is stimulated, i.e. starts when oxygen absorbtion falls below a critical value. Now a very important factor for the regeneration process is the demand for oxygen and substances that can be oxydized.

This is where the essential fatty acids are now a desicive factor – as I demonstrated 1951/52 – in restoring the harmony in the redox system, particularly for oxygen absorbtion in the cytochrome system. Then in the subsequent wound healing, in the process of regeneration in which cell division is accelerated, this process is nevertheless controlled by the superordinate regulating system in the body. Autonomous, unlimited growth does not take place.

To summarize: In the highly unsaturated fatty acids I found a substance which is capable of influencing the immature division, particularly in cancer cells, with the desired effect that this substance does not have a harmful influence on normal cells and the vital functions. This substance restores the harmony in the disturbed organism.

It is the conviction of the author that this suggested avenue of research affords the shortest path to cure cancer, and to overcome it. Today it is a burning necessity to draw the practical consequences. This is also a burning necessity for established cancer research. Scientific and humanitarian considerations demand this course correction.

This manuscript with introduction has been submitted to the Carolinska Medico Kirurgiska Institut in Stockholm in English. The author was nominated for the Nobel Prize for medicine by representatives of the medical community in Germany and in other countries.

1.) New directions in fat analysis.

I opened new ways of fat analysis through the development of paper chromatography of fats (1950). This meant that for the first time, fats, fatty acids, and lipoproteides could be detected directly and in the smallest proportions, and thus characterized and studied in the form of microanalysis. For example using Co 60 I was successful in producing the first differentiation reaction between oil and linolenic acid, and via radioiodine producing the first direct iodine value. Original studies in this area are published in "Oil & Soap". Compilations are in "Photo elements of life" (1979) and in the "Fat Syndrome" (1959), as well as in "The elementary function of respiration in its relationship to autoxydable nutrients".

The presence and harmful effects of the polymerized fats highly unsaturated fatty acids in the poly oils were proven and confirmed in animal experiments (1951). Correspondence in this regard with the Ministry of Food is present as is the publication (1952). ,

2.) New biological findings regarding the highly unsaturated fatty acids rich in pi-electrons in lipoids.

I recognized and proved the significance of cis linoleic acid in the function of respiratory enzymes for the first time. The linoleic acid as partner to the sulfhydryl group as creator of the lipoproteins was recognized, proven and discussed in its fundamental important effect for each vital function (1952). I discussed the electromotoric function of the pi electrons of the highly unsaturated linoleic acid in the lipoid membrane in the microstructure of protoplasm, for all nerve functions, secretions, mitosis, as well as cell break-down, in this context.

Torsten Thunberg wrote in 1951 in the manual ("B. Flaschenträger"): Here the entire problem of medicine reaches its summit "to find the great unknown", the second pair of the sulfhydryl group in the autoxydable system of the cell. Linoleic acid proved to be this "great unknown".

In his attempts to re-stimulate oxidation, which was suppressed through tumor formation, **O. Warburg** had assumed that a fatty acid must play a role in this process. His attempts to achieve this with butyric acid or coconut acid failed. He did not want to interpret this so "unexpected reversal. Here I now use the highly unsaturated cis-linoleic acid, rich in pi electrons as the crucial factor. The oxidation processes are normalized.

This applies for the lipoid membrane of the cell. It was confirmed and photographically recorded (1953) for the lipoid membrane of the erythrocytes. This is what is missing in the case of cancer illness, the lipoid membrane and its electromotoric effect.

Ivar Bang who did extensive work on the significance of the lipoid membrane (1911) wrote that it could be a fatty acid that plays a role here. This is autoxydable, sensitive to light. "It is not oleic acid". While Ivar Bang considered the integrity of the lipoid membrane to be crucial for all vital functions he combines this etiologically with the occurrence and overcoming of carcinomas. (1911). What was missing was a verification method for linoleic acid.

Hans von Euler, Stockholm in 1949 cited "separation of fat" as the common denominator for all tumor types, where it is not normally present as lipoid. For instance, the function of the highly unsaturated fats as partner of the sulfhydryl group also overcomes the separation of the fats in the blood!

A.I. Virtanen, Helsinki, agreed with my comments in Basel 1952, he stated that he had observed that the increased accumulation of fats in the cell is one criterion for the inactivity of the lipoids in their function. It is obstructively noticeable – and this applies to all the research regarding lipoids and lipoproteides – that a detection method for highly unsaturated linoleic acid to this date, 1951 was not present.

My application of the new analytical method for examining the blood lipoids in the native stage from a drop of blood on paper resulted, among other things, in an important detection method for cancer, also for tumor formation in the initial stages, which thus could not yet be detected through radiology (in this regard see the article published in 1952 in "Oil & Soap" as well as the fig. in the "Fat Syndrome" 1959 Table II Fig. c, d, e.).

Experiments on this cytochrome tail, which is positive for cancer via gamma portions of the linoleic acid, were revealing. 1/1000mg of linoleic added to the drop of blood inhibits the criteria that are typical for cancer. To this day these verifications of cancer are still more certain and more simple than radiological verifications.

Then in 1953, I undertook the localization of this finding in native blood with a 2-phase contrast microscope! This was done with healthy individuals and sick individuals also using the oil-protein diet.

The results, briefly summarized:

The pairing of the sulfhydryl group for all cell-constituting substances with cis-linoleic acid, possibly combined with linolenic acid, which is more rich in electrons, are substances of high physiological interest for all vital functions.

The labil hydrogen of the sulfhydryl group, in association with the energy rich pi-electron systems of the cis-linoleic acid or linolenic acid, or other polyunsaturated fatty acids, produces the prerequisite for the hydrogen bridge of the lipoproteide with elevated energy level, which is essential for all electron exchanges in the living substrate.

The Bohr frequency conditions for absorbtion or emission of light quanta, the photons, are present in this hydrogen, to transfer the electronic energy of the pi electrons to protein (changing the energy level).

These substances, which are of high physiological interest, they are autoxydable sensitive to light, they store and conduct photons, they have a high affinity for oxygen and high electromagnetic force relative to the absorbtion of solar energy, must be constantly re-supplied and kept functional through the unsatureated fats with their pi electrons found in foodstuffs. This function of the highly unsaturated fats, fatty acids, lechithins including lipoids with high spreading effect with their large surface activity was studied through paper chromotography, then it was also studied iin the native blood under the 2-phase contrast microscope, e.g. on the lipoid membrane of the erythrocytes, (I was the first person to use it in blood). The lipid layer of the highly unsaturated fatty acids also proved to be significant with reference to lipoid replenishment in the living human skin.

3.) The function of the pi electrons of the fatty acids in accordance with electron biology.

I drew on electron biology to extend the newly acquired insights concerning the significance of the highly unsaturated fatty acids for the biology of the lipoid membrane, fat metabolism for respiration, protein build up and mitosis for growth processes. The diene (pi electrons) act as bases in the extended sense of the word.

The possibility thus recognized for controlling the redox potential, also makes it possible bring the metabolism of the highly unsaturated fats in combination with the biological immune processes of the lymph system. This affects the immunobiological processes for all defense against illness, for secretions, in particularly the membrane functions of the kidneys, liver, prostate, the stomach and of the pancreas, as well as control of the sexual functions (see "Fat Syndrome" 1959).

In accordance with electron biology the result is that the cis form of the fatty acids is always more rich in energy. On the other hand, the effect of the transforms promotes the tendency to lack of energy, acts against the increased energy level of the pi-electron cloud of the polyene. This also applies for polymerisates of the fats, used as emulgents.

The polyene compound acts as oscillator for the electron energy. This affects the entire pi-electron cloud, the intensity of the absorption with preference for the longest wavelengths of the light.

Inclusion Niels Bohr's work regarding the energy level of hydrogen electrons is significant for the function of the hydrogen bridge, and of the lipoproteides from the highly unsaturaged fatty acids and the sulfhydryl group. In the quantum energy exchange in the biological system the hydrogen bridge is considered as the only location for the rapid and aligned energy exchange energy in the biological system. In this context the possibility of controlling, raising, this electromotoric force via the pi-electrons of the unsaturated fats and lipoids, is of crucial significance as anti-entropy factor for all processes of the vital function, particularly for the lipoids on all membranes.

The accretion of the electromotoric force of the liproteides, of the pi-electrons in the lipoid membranes, can be evaluated not only according to the number of pi-electrons. This can also be viewed relatively, e.g. to the length of the polyene chain. Thus the triple unsaturated bond of the linolenic acid (octodecatrien acid) is more intensively effective than a quadruple bond of a polyene compound with 20 or 26 links for example. In this process however other related substances like carotene, vitamin E, or in the opposite sense preservative substance must be taken into consideration. The elevated stimulation condition of the polyene also affects the proton affinity, the tendency to form pi-complexes, for instance with metals. The activation energy of the pi-electron cloud decisively influences the resonance energy.

This resonance, the quantum interaction when exchanging forces affects not only the different arrangement possibilities within the systems, pi-electron cloud, hydrogen bridge, associates, function of the membrane in substance transport and energy transport. These resonance processes can be strongly influenced by the external effect of electrical and magnetic fields, through photons.

As far as I know, I was the first to recognize and work out this interaction between photons and pi-electrons, which in its function still allows the heritage of its forebears, the quanta of solar energy to be recognized. I published these relationships on the international level, e.g. they were presented in my book. "Laser rays against cancer" (1968) also documented in the book "Der Tod des Tumors" Band II "Die Dokumentation" (The death of the Tumor Vol. II The Documentation).

4. The quantum biology of the pi-electron cloud in the highly unsaturated systems.

The newly detected cardinal function of the highly unsaturated fats as foodstuff is clearly evident for man in membranes but also as components of plasma. This applies particularly when the whole thing is viewed from the quantum biological perspective. The physicist Erwin Schrödinger sought the "anti-entropy factor" for the vital function of the human being. The synergy of the pi-electrons of the fats and the solar energy photons allows this "anti entropy factor" of the vital function of the human being to be detected.

With his work on the radiation capacity of matter, the physicist Louie de Broglie supplied good calculations on the dualism of light between light and matter. The beautiful physical treatment of the functions of photons provided by the physicist Kenneth W. Ford (see "The World of Elementary Particles") emphasized quantum electrodynamics for the function of electrons and photons as fundamental interaction, as elementary events of all interactions in nature.

My work was the first to specify these "events of fundamental significance" based on fat metabolism, the pi-electrons with the solar energy photons.

The fundamental considerations of **Kenneth W. Ford** on being human and "anti-mensch" allow us to recognize the framework in which my work on the pi-electrons of the highly unsaturated fats, and resonance with solar energy should be viewed.

The sunlight integrated in the vital function of the human being via the essential fats, lipoids represents such an elementary fundamental vital function that disturbances at this point affect plainly affect the human being. The dynamics of all membrane functions are borne by these lipoids. The light of the sun, essential for the vital function of the human being is attracted, absorbed, conducted, stored in depots, and as quantum discontinually arranged by the force of the solar electrons, the pi-electron systems as energy in the vital processes, ad "anti-entropy factor".

The photon does not age. Time stands still for the photon due to the power of its speed of light. In the interplay with matter, the living substance, this photon transfers a high energy level, in interaction with the pi-electrons, to the high degree of organization for man, for being human. Clouds of photons in the pi-electron cloud transfer something of the nature of light to the living substance of the human being. According to **Friedrich Dessauer** the human being can store more solar energy than other life forms can.

Light promotes evolution. A deficency in photons in living substance hinders evolution. It promotes the development of an "anti-mensch" (according to **Feynmann**). The quantum allocation remains essential for energy distribution. The pi-electrons of the highly unsaturated fats as quanta correspond to the photons of the sun. The events of this fundamental interaction can by represented by computable diagrams. They affect the high level of organization of the human being. The fascinating role of the photon, of light in the basic system of the human being becomes clear in the framework of these considerations. It is also clear how extensively the disturbance is, which on broader level via edible fats, feed products in the production of meat and preservatives of food-stuffs via chemicals disrupts and hinders the function of the pi-electrons in interaction with solar energy.

The progress of natural science cannot disregard these elemental issues of the creation. The gentle substance of the wave fields, solarized, compressed in the pi-electrons of fats is essential for the vital function, also for overcoming the formation of tumors.

5.) The practical appplication

The practical application of these findings on pi-electrons e.g. fatty acids in their synergism with the photons of sunlight is simple and successful. It is also successful for cancer patients. The realization of this idea is structured in such a manner that growth-promoting vitamins, lecithins and metal complexes support the function of the highly unsaturated fats in interplay with sulphur-containing protein support. The sun is used preferetially, also Eldi oil is applied externally to promote the absorbtion of the sun in the long-wave ranges. (Eldi oils - Electron Differential oils - contain pi-electron clouds of the linoleic acids and linolinic acids as well as vitamin E in natural structure, aether oils and sulfydryl group). Radiation and substances which have a disassociating effect on the association of fat and protein are avoided. These are narcotically acting substances, often pain-relieving substances. These are avoided because they disturb the build-up of energy and the function of the lipoid membrane. Practical application of the oils internally and externally truly allows extensive deactivation of narcotic substances.

The observed practical effects of the this oil-protein cure:

With **lymphogranulomatosis** success occurs quickly, it is relatively certain, and sustainable over 10, or even 20 year.

For tumors in the **prostate** or in the **breast**, the tumor is often dissolved or eliminated within a few weeks. This aid is even possible after cytostatic treatment and in the presence of metastatsis.

The effect of this oil-protein cure for **brain tumors** in the lateral ventricle of the brain is very surprising. Usually the separation of the tumor and elimination is recognizable for the patients and family via the nose / throat area. This aid is sustainable i.e. when complying with the basic principles in accordance with the preceding guidelines. Additional tumors or metastasis do not occur.

For **leukemia** the success with children is fast and clear. The nutrition-based cause is quite noticiable here. For older persons with leukemia and tumor in the spleen, success is not so fast, but it is clear.

It suffices to list these examples: For science the guideline should be to promote growth forces, to overcome the jam that is associated with tumor formation.

Hans von Euler determined that foreign fats are recognizable as common denomiator for **all types of tumors**. All cancer noxa unfold their characterisitic as cancer noxa only if they are released in fats, particularly in "bad fats". Fats that are rich in pi-electrons in association with the sulfydryl group in the plasma and in membranes, overcome the separation of fats that are foreign to the body. They overcome the effect of benzpyrene and cancer noxa.

6). My path of scientific proof

In 1951 as senior expert for fats and medication I worked concurrently:
a) on the function of "lipotropic" medications;
b) on the analysis for characterizing fats and fatty acids.

I noticed: in the medical world the type of fat of the lipo itself was not considered in scientific studies on "lipotropic" substances. In 1951 my experiment (see Fat Syndrome Table 1 Fig. c) proved the adhesion of the sulfhydryl group with the diene fatty acid and the impact of solubility of fats.

A year went by until I with Professor K. could publish these scientific findings, the theoretical work substantiated with practical proofs. A lot of resistance was noticiable. Indeed in 1952 when I refused the offer from Professor K. not to publish anything else in exchange for hush money, I did not fully appreciate the associated risk. I lost my job, and any other possibility to work in an institute was also obstructed. However my decision was correct in the service of the truth of cience.

In my efforts, in collaboration with clinics, to put realization to the test, I always found friends but also found bitter counter-actions. The major capital of the Unilever margarine industry would appear now and again sporadically and legally tangible. This was associated with the disruption of my medical studies. In this context Prof. M. in Göttingen put an end to his own life.

In my own practice I realize here these findings. The major involvement of capital from the Unilever industry, and "experts" was also legally tangible here. "The lust for gold produces incurable confusion in people's heads" stated Las Casis before Carl V in his efforts against the slave trade. It is the same today. Incurable confusion is used in the press relative to the fat issue. Those who control this press are very well aware that there is a difference between the "linolenic acid with active pi-electrons in natural form, and the "linolenic acid" that is stabilized, deformed, deactivated, for instance with trans linolenic acids.

It is part of the nobility of pure science that those who pursue never take their eyes off of utilization for good. It is considered wisdom in science to decide for the correct practical application.

7.) Summary of the science of the highly unsaturated fats for the dynamics in the life process.

The crucial threshold layer of the living substance is the lipoid membrane. Its energy condition is descisive for the electromotoric force of the vital function. The hemolytic effect of x-rays on the erythrocytes is based on the change of the protein lipoid hull (**Fr. Dessauer**).

Restoration of the damaged lipid layer on the erythrocytes succeeds through administration of the oil-protein diet, and is a cardinal point for the restoration of the lipoid membrane as criterion of the vital function. The occurrence of cramp symptoms and of carcinomas after x-rays and the opposite effect of the pi-electrons show the large framework of entropy processes and anti-entropy effect in which both must be viewed here; on one hand entropy and death-facilitation through x-rays, on the other hand the function of pi-electrons as antenna for solar energy as vital element, as photo element of life, as anti-entropy factor of life.

Everything that deepens the potential cavity in the energy balance of the vital function through mutation, deactivation of the flow balance in the metabolism, hinders the electron exchange, promotes entropy in the life process also, and favors the occurrence of carcinomas.

Everything that raises the energy balance of the solar pi-electrons, supports their quantum transport, discontinually as needed, fills their energy depot, raises the potential of vital energy, works against cancer.

In modern physics the knowledge of the electron was extended in an unexpected manner by the discovery of the wave characteristic of the electron. The science of electromagnetism brought great progress to technology. It now represents an essential element, applied to biological problems to also teach us to master the cause and overcome the occurrence of cancer. The relativistic dynamics of the electron can now be integrated in the vital process of the human being via the pi-electrons of the highly unsaturated fats, arranged to the sun from a quantum perspective.

The physical-chemical structure of the pi-electron clouds in the lipoid membrane, with their effects on the electromotoric field forces in metabolism, and for photon absorption, for the storage of solar energy, represents such a significant prerequisite for the vital function that the comments of Ivar Bang prove true:

Fats are governing substances of all vital functions.

Below there are a few sentences of the American physician Dr. Jan Roehm who studied my therapy intensively.

"I wish that all my students had the education of a biochemist and quantum physicist so that they could understand the perfect composition of this diet. It is a miracle. The idea with the champagne is so easy to accpet and can get people out off of their death bed. An enema with 250 ml of oil is another life-extending way through that electron-rich oil gets into the body. It can also be rubbed on the skin and gets into the body through the skin.

You should follow this diet for app. 5 years. After this time your tumor should disappear completely. The condition of people who have stopped the diet too soon (by eating meat and candy) worsens quickly and these people cannot be saved after such a bodily torture.

Cancer treatment could be very simple and very successful if one knows how. But the interests of the cancer industry are not lined up to allow you to have this knowledge. May those who are ill with cancer (including you and your friends) forgive the heavyweights, for keeping this simple information unavailable to you for so long."

Basis of my nutritional advice

As an example for the basis of my nutritional advice for the oil-protein diet, I would like to add a guideline for starting with my nutrition guideline. This guideline is modified is initialy adapted to the sick person or normal consumer. Also my counsel is extended over time relative to the situation on trips, on vacation, or for social events.

In conjunction with the change in diet, my consultation also includes the use of ELDI oils externally, as well as ELDI oil enemas.

These consultations should be executed by a specialist who also has knowledge of the significance of the electromagnetic field in the sick person's environment.

Nutrition guideline

For starting the oil-protein diet

1-2-3 transition days: depending on the prescription:

( ) Oatmeal with Linomel cereal every hour
( ) Oatmeal soup with Linomel 3x daily
( ) 250 g Linomel * daily with juices, as prescribed
Ferment gold (papaya juice) is very important.
10:00 - carrot juice, fresh pressed

Ensure that you take a warm drink at least 3 x a day e.g. green tea or herbal tea. Sweeten it only with honey. Seriously ill patients also do well with this transition!

Oil-protein diet from the _____ day on.

7:00   1 glass of sauerkraut juice.

8:00   Breakfast: 1 glass of tea e.g. green tea, possibly with honey, then the Linomel muesli:

* **Linomel** is a flaxseed / honey mixture - only available in Germany. An alternative is **fresh** grounded flaxseed.

2 spoonfuls of Linomel with fruit start with a grated apple. then layer quark-flax oil crème according to the guideline above also with added flavoring. Add the flavoring in drops.

The Linomel muesli

1 tsp honey
3 tblsp milk
3 tblsp flax seed oil
100 g Quark
2 tblsp Linomel or fresh
ground flaxseeds as an
alternative
Fresh fruits and fruit juices
nuts

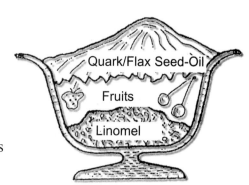

10:00-11:00: Fresh-pressed juices Carrot juice, radish juice, stinging nettle juice, with lemon, as prescribed.

Info: Create your own Oleolux

12:00 PM 1 tablespoon Linomel, 1 glass of champagne

12:15 PM Appetizer:
Salad plate with quark-flaxseed mayonnaise.
As salad also use: Dandelion, cress, celery, lambs lettuce, radish, sauerkraut, horseradish, green pepper,
for mayonnaise use:

Quark, flax oil, milk, lemon herbal salt,
possibly mustard, sour pickle, garlic,
in addition a lot of herbs, fresh or dried.

12:30 PM   Main dish Vegetables cooked in water,
then flavored with Oleolux and
herbs possibly with oatmeal
soy sauce, curry etc.

Vegetable broth flavored with a little
Oleolux and yeast flakes,
(serve heartily seasoned as bouillon).

As side dish for the vegetables:
a) buckwheat, standard recipe (boiled like
    rice)
b) buckwheat according to the cookbook
c) brown rice, millet
d) potatoes boiled in the peel. potatoes
    as mashed potatoes (prepared with Oleolux
    and milk).

Desert: Quark-flax oil cream with honey;
mixed with fresh fruit, and real vanilla and/or
1-teaspoon vodka, rum, cherry or plum
brandy.

3:00 PM   1 tablespoon Linomel, 1 glass champagne or
1teaspoon Linomel and 1 glass grape juice or
muscatel cherry or pineapple juice.

3:30   1 tablespoon Linomel, 1 – 3 glasses of pure
              juice (Pure ruby, pure saphire, cherry pure
              juice, pure blueberry juice). or papaya juice.

6:00 PM   Soup made of buckwheat groats in vegetable
              broth, well seasoned, flavor with Oleolux
              Add 1 teaspoon of yeast flakes.

8.30 PM   1 glass of red wine, possibly with some
              honey.

Oleolux Recipe

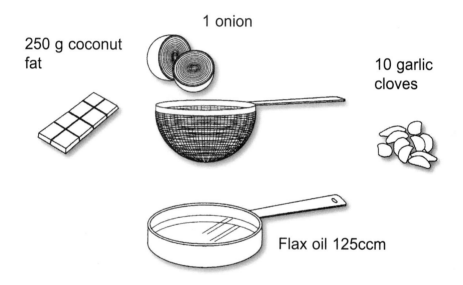

250 g coconut fat

1 onion

10 garlic cloves

Flax oil 125ccm

Cut one medium sized onion in half and brown slightly in 250 g of heated coconut fat. Cook for appr. 15 minutes and add 10 garlic cloves and heat for additional 3 minutes. Strain the fat through a sieve into 125ccm of flax seed oil (previously chilled for 30 minutes in the freeze). Keep this mixture always refrigerated.

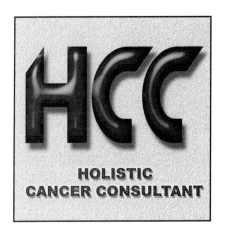

HOLISTIC CANCER CONSULTANT

An introduction to a new vocational profile

Independent, holistic cancer consulting

Sooner or later all those who are involved intensively with non-conventional cancer therapies, are confronted with the same problem: The majority of all patients only turn to biological therapies when conventional therapies have failed. Unfortunately the starting point at which a biological therapy is employed is totally different than it was when chemotherapy or irradiation was administered, because our body is no longer the same after irradiation or chemotherapy, not even if "objective data", such as hemograms, stabilize after several weeks.

In 99.9% of cases cancer is diagnosed by conventionally trained physicians, and consequently most patients are also treated conventionally. However, since doctors are only slightly familiar (or not at all familiar) with non-conventional therapies (mistletoe, thymus, enzymes, vitamins, etc.), and often they still have a large information deficit concerning the statistics on conventionally used therapies, patients usually can only choose between an operation, chemotherapy, and irradiation.

The greatest deficit however with those directly affected, and this also includes family members, who usually are not in a situation where they can make rational decisions immediately after the diagnosis. The emotional involvement does not permit this. This is unfortunately the reason why far too many rash decisions are still being made; decisions that many patients later regret. This is understandable, because when people have cancer, they almost always believe that they do not have any time to consider things, or to research the issues.

But let's be honest:

* what doctor provides his patients with copies of studies about the chemotherapy or the irradiation that will be administered?

* What doctor is even capable of describing a conventional approach AND a non-conventional approach?

* what patient can pose THE questions to his doctor that are really important (due to the patient's lack of knowledge and the emotional impact of the patient's diagnosis)?

However it particularly these three points that are the most important after a diagnosis of cancer. Unfortunately there are only a few people who have the good fortune to be able to sit across the table from a doctor who is familiar with both important directions of oncology. Another major challenge is to determine whether the therapy offered would help just the patient, or whether it also helps others. For a number of very different reasons many patients are "directed into studies" and thus they lose forever the chance that is afforded by non-conventional, successful, therapies. On the other hand others pay for expensive non-conventional therapies and only determine much too late that the therapies offered do not even come close to being worth the money. Unfortunately the issues of money, career, and therapies are almost always related and thus it is very difficult for a lay person (and often for experts as well) to understand whether the therapies offered are independent from other – mostly financial – interests. This is the reason why other teachers and I started offering career training to those interested in becoming a holistic cancer consultant.

FAQ

How do we do this?

We train people to be consultants, not therapists (consultants are people who only advise cancer patients verbally; they do not perform any therapy, not even psychological therapy. Therapists are people who use therapies on patients, or with patients). We consider separation between treating specialist/therapist and consultant to be absolutely necessary so that conflicts of interest do not even occur. This is the only that a patient can be 100 % certain that he is being advised independently. A consultant earns money with his work, but ONLY with his verbal work, he does not earn "supplemental income" which unfortunately is the status quo today. Naturally we make all of our knowledge available to our consultants, this particularly includes which doctors and clinics offer holistic treatment, or successfully treat cancer.

May I request money for my consulting later?

Of course. Every holistic cancer consultant can and should advise people based on his personal life context (self-help group leader, former patient, physician, psychologist, naturopath, etc.), and naturally he should also be paid for this advice. The only difference between a treating specialist and the consultant is that the consultant does not perform any therapy on his own, for which he receives money from patients.

How long is the training course?

You can make the course online and is depending how much time you are investing.

What does the training course include?

An extensive curriculum in which the minimum knowledge required to holistically advise people with cancer is presented. Naturally this also includes the entire 3E program (Eat healthy, Eliminate toxins, Energetic work) and the knowledge of different cancer therapies, standard allopathic therapies, and diagnosis, and most importantly, knowledge of which conventional and non-conventional therapies are demonstrably successful for which types of cancer. The training enables each consult to create a consulting offering for his work. We do not think that each consultant should work in the same manner. Just as each patient is a unique individual, so each consultant must identify for himself the best way that he can advise and accompany people who are ill. We regard this point as the greatest challenge of the training course.

Do I need basic medical knowledge?

Yes and no. Basically we say that natural medical training will be quite helpful in learning the material, however it is not a necessity, if the person being trained is prepared to acquire the necessary knowledge.

Who are the instructors?

Mr. Lothar Hirneise, and others who can contribute to achieving the learning objective.

Please describe the activity of a holistic cancer consultant in practical terms?

Naturally the answer to these questions depends on the context of the individual, the professional experience of the individual, or the profession in which the individual would like to work. Basically the consultants offer accompaniment on the patient's path – regardless of whether the patient wants to pursue a conventional path, or a non-conventional path. The consulting can take a few hours (3E program, accompanying the patient to the oncologist etc.) or it can extend over a longer period. Also close collaboration with the treating therapist is possible.

Where can I be trained and how much does it cost?

Up to this point the training was only available in Germany. Currently in Europe there are trained cancer consultants, or cancer consultants in training, in Germany, Austria, France, Holland, Slovenia, and in Spain. From summer 2010 you can make the course online. More information: nexusgmbh@t-online.de

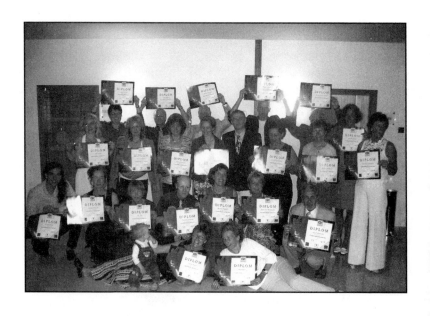

HCC graduating class 2005 in Mallorca / Spain

In the future there will be two groups of cancer patients. Those who have read this book - and those who are uninformed.

For many years Lothar Hirneise has been traveling throughout the world looking for the most successful cancer therapies, and he has been explaining to people that there is much more available than just chemotherapy and irradiation. Recognized internationally as Europe's leading specialist in this area, he describes the results of his years of research in this encyclopedia of non-conventional therapies. The reader will also learn in detail why so-called experts in reality know little about cancer. In addition to descriptions of more than 100 cancer therapies and substances used in treating cancer, the author also explains which cancer therapies are used allopathically, for which types of cancer, and what is imperative for a patient to know before he subjects himself to such therapies.

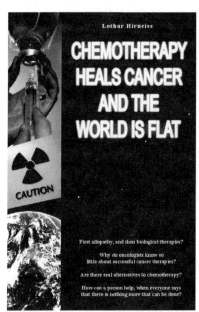

The 3E program, which is based on the analysis of case histories of thousands of people who have survived late stage cancer, is also described for the first time, Learn why so many people die of cancer, and why so many others do not. This book not only supplies an incredible amount of information, it also helps the cancer patient to find his own way to cure cancer through the active exercises of the 3E program.

772 pages!

www.nexus-book.com

Coming soon:

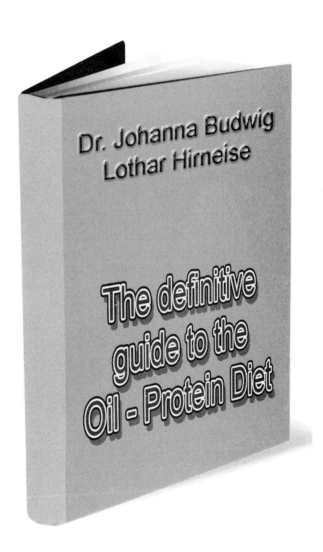

Dr. Johanna Budwig
Lothar Hirneise

The definitive
guide to the
Oil - Protein Diet

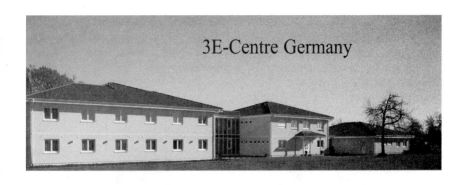
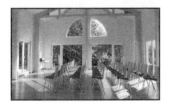
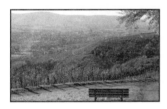
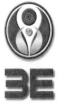
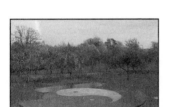
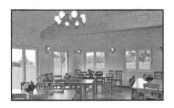

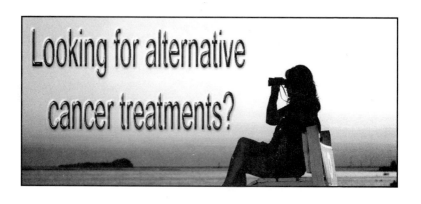

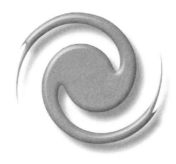

CANCER 21

THE 21ST CENTURY ONCOLOGY

www.cancer-21.com